GINKGO A

GINKGO AND GARLIC

Natural Remedies for Respiratory and Circulatory Problems

Nicola Peterson

SOUVENIR PRESS

First published 1998 by
Souvenir Press Ltd,
43 Great Russell Street, London WC1B 3PA

ISBN 0 285 63432 1

Typeset by Rowland Phototypesetting Ltd,
Bury St Edmunds, Suffolk

Printed in Great Britain by
The Guernsey Press Company Ltd,
Guernsey, Channel Islands

This book is dedicated to
the spirit of respect and co-operation
between the scientific community and herbal medicine
which is coming into being and will flourish
with due nurturing

Acknowledgement

My husband, Roger McFadden, deserves to be credited as co-author of this book. I am indebted to him for spending more hours than he could spare researching and formulating the ideas for the last two chapters of the book. Also for providing me with healthy and delicious meals every night of the week.

Note to Readers

The aim of this book is to provide information on the uses of ginkgo and garlic in the treatment of relevant diseases. Although every care has been taken to ensure that the advice is accurate and practical, it is not intended to be a guide to self-diagnosis and self-treatment. Where health is concerned—and in particular a serious problem of any kind—it must be stressed that there is no substitute for seeking advice from a qualified medical practitioner. All persistent symptoms, of whatever nature, may have underlying causes that need, and should not be treated without, professional elucidation and evaluation.

It is therefore very important, if you are considering trying ginkgo and garlic, to consult your practitioner first, and if you are already taking any prescribed medication, do not stop it.

The Publisher makes no representation, express or implied, with regard to the accuracy of the information contained in this book, and legal responsibility or liability cannot be accepted by the Author or the Publisher for any errors or omissions that may be made or for any loss, damage, injury or problems suffered or in any way arising from following the advice offered in these pages.

Contents

Preface

Twenty years ago, when I started my training to become a herbal practitioner, the subject was thought to be very 'fringe' and odd. I was attracted to it because, having an interest in botany, I was intrigued by the idea of using plants medicinally, and the more I learned the more inspired I became. Since then the experience of sixteen years in practice has confirmed my confidence in the value of herbal medicine for many people whom other types of treatment have not helped. At the start this was against a background of general scepticism from most doctors, although not from the general public. I like to compare this attitude with the current climate of orthodox medical opinion in Europe. If you consult a doctor in Germany or France with a problem such as hardening of the arteries, angina or memory impairment due to deficiency of the circulation, you will probably be prescribed a herb. The doctor may not think of it as such, because it is a remedy that has been put through extensive clinical trials and is in the form of a standard-dose tablet. But basically you will be prescribed a type of leaf.

Recognising the extensive use of both ginkgo and garlic by orthodox doctors in Europe, this book has been written in the anticipation of growing interest in these herbs in the UK. This will come from both lay people interested in keeping themselves healthy, and from health professionals in orthodox and complementary medicine. My intention is not to give an account of the professional herbalist's approach to the treatment of circulatory and respiratory problems, but to provide accurate information on the remedies in two ways: firstly, in Part One, to lay people, with explanations of how heart and circulation problems develop, and how they can be tackled with changes in exercise, dietary regimes, and the use of garlic and ginkgo, and secondly, in Part Two, to professionals who are interested in up-to-date research.

N. P.

CHAPTER 1

How Ginkgo and Garlic Can Help You

Your first thought on seeing the title of this book might well be, 'Why ginkgo and garlic?' What do these two species, one a little-known Chinese tree and the other a smelly Mediterranean bulb, have in common? The answer is that, despite being different in practically every respect, they can be used together to improve the health of just about everyone who is at risk from the diseases of our modern way of life.

We in the West have much to be thankful for. Our technically advanced society represents the most affluent and labour-free mass culture in human history, and the scientific and technical developments of the recent past have led us to imagine a future in which everything will get better and better. However, we now know that there is a price to pay for the richer (but more polluted and less active) way of life we have adopted. Our bodies are not well adapted to it, and certain illnesses that were rare a few generations ago have become the modern epidemics. Heart and blood-vessel diseases, known collectively as 'cardiovascular disease', which include coronary heart disease and stroke, are now responsible for the majority of deaths in the United Kingdom each year. The two most important factors behind this increase are changes in exercise and eating habits. There has been a reduction in the average amount of exercise that people take compared with previous generations, and a change in diet away from fruit, vegetables and traditional cooking methods towards high-fat, high-sugar fast foods.

The proliferation in cases of childhood asthma may also be

associated with our growing affluence. Studies point to an increased exposure in our present-day houses to substances likely to provoke allergic reactions. Central heating and wall-to-wall carpets provide the ideal conditions in which dust mites breed, and if young children are exposed to a high level of them in early life, their immune systems may become 'programmed' to react to them in later childhood in the form of asthma. High levels of air pollution may further aggravate this, after the reaction has become established. Here too diet is thought to be a factor, as the peak time for the development of new cases of asthma in the 1980s coincided with the period at which fruit and vegetable consumption by the population was at its lowest. Since then, health education policies have had some success in getting across the message that we all need at least two pieces of fruit and three portions of vegetables every day to stay healthy.

Perhaps the acknowledgement of the nutritional benefits of vegetables has stimulated interest in their therapeutic potential. Research is revealing that numerous previously unknown substances, referred to as *phytonutrients* (meaning dietary components that are found only in plants and are essential for good health) abound in the most humble fruit and vegetables, and have a wealth of protective influences on our health. It takes only a small step in thought to extend the investigation to plants that have until recently been regarded as the province of fringe medicine.

Some people find it astonishing that plants can provide our medicines as well as our food. This is a view characteristic only of technological Western cultures; in most other parts of the world, plants have always been the main source of food, medicine, and often, raw materials for the manufacture of essential artefacts. The World Health Organisation is keen to help traditional cultures maintain their knowledge of local medicinal plants: they are easily accessible and affordable, whereas imported drug treatments may be neither. The loss of plant species due to increasing use of land for agriculture poses a threat to local wild plants, and conservation projects in many endangered areas are targeting the preservation of medicinal plants. In contrast, the cultivation of plants like garlic and ginkgo, which are of accepted medicinal value in the West, is expanding because of their guaranteed commercial worth.

Ginkgo biloba, otherwise known as the maidenhair tree because of the similarity of its leaves to those of the maidenhair fern, is a native of China. Until recently it has been familiar only to botanists and gardeners, appreciated for the beauty of its form and its unique botanical niche. Garlic, however, has long been known to all— loved by some, loathed by others for the aroma it imparts to food and to the breath of those who eat it. Ginkgo is a tree of grace and distinction, but requires patience on the part of those who wish to cultivate it—its growth rate is such that one gardener's advice is to 'plant it for the delight of your grandchildren'. This holds true for more distant generations as well, because some ginkgos alive today are thought to have been planted around one thousand years ago. However, if garlic is your aim, you can have a mature and rewarding crop by planting single cloves, split from the clump that forms the whole corm, in early autumn, and harvesting them ten months later. Though less aesthetically pleasing than ginkgo, the sight of a strong and healthy row or two of garlic plants bring satisfaction to innumerable enthusiastic gardeners.

The chemical constituents of the two plants are very different. All plants are remarkable natural chemical 'factories', and produce an enormous number of different substances from the very basic raw materials that they take in from the soil and air. They build these simple substances into complex ones by harvesting and using the energy in sunlight, and thus have a range of constituents far greater than any animal species produces in its body. These will help them survive in their own particular (sometimes inhospitable) environment. It is not surprising, therefore, that ginkgo, being a tree with its home in China, should make a different range of substances from garlic, which is a biennial plant thought to have originated in south-west Siberia. What is more remarkable is that several of the constituents of both plants have a striking therapeutic effect on the human circulatory and respiratory systems.

However, without the information that has been revealed through modern research, the benefits of many plants would be known only to those who, like myself, have chosen to study herbal medicine. The subject has been opened up enormously by research that is acceptable to orthodox as well as natural practitioners, and I hope it will lead to a better understanding between the two. Science has discovered and named over eighteen thousand different *phytochemicals* (plant chemicals), each family of plants not only having its own unique combination but also individual chemicals unique to that family. Many of these are produced as defences against insects and fungi, others are intermediates in biochemical pathways; but for the vast majority, their function is unknown to science.

Research has certainly validated the traditional uses of both garlic and ginkgo in cardiovascular and respiratory disease. An idea of the recent amount of interest in these plant medicines is given by the fact that in the last ten years there have been hundreds of research papers published on ginkgo, and in 1990 alone there were 2,000 published on garlic. Scientifically respectable journals such as the *Lancet* and the *American Journal of Medicine* have published articles on both of them. In Germany, where the use of herbal remedies has always been popular with the public, but where there has also been stringent official investigation, garlic was the best-selling remedy until 1991, when it was overtaken by ginkgo. Doctors' prescriptions for it there make it one of the largest-selling treatments for circulatory problems. In the UK 10 per cent of the population take garlic for its medicinal benefit.

Why do so many people use these remedies? The answer, as we have seen, is that cardiovascular disease and asthma are on the increase. Although fewer people today experience the infectious epidemic diseases of the past, and although we are much more likely to recover from accidental injury, our way of life results in us being vulnerable to these other serious problems. Asthma may start in childhood, but the slow deterioration of the circulation may not become apparent until middle age. There can be disabling problems with both diseases that limit people's quality of life well before they can be considered to be old. Of course there are life-saving drugs available, but while these are prolonging the lives of sick people, they are not always able to restore a good quality of life. Now that we are all much more likely to live longer than previous generations, we need to give more thought in our youth to how to preserve our health into older age, so that the extra years can be a blessing rather than a trial. Advice to the public about healthy lifestyles is one aspect of this. The use of helpful natural supplements that can be taken safely for long periods of time— that can in fact be thought of as a regular component of a healthy dietary regime—is another. By taking garlic and ginkgo people are trying to halt the damage and prevent the serious consequences of advanced disease. So in the late twentieth century these remedies have come into their own.

Garlic must be one of the most universal of plant medicines, used in the majority of human cultures and at most times throughout recorded history. From its home in south-west Siberia it spread to the Middle East. The first known prescription dates back to 3000 BC, in the Sumerian civilisation. Fifteen hundred years later there is a reference to it in an Egyptian medical papyrus. It was well known to the ancient Greeks, being popular with them as a food, as medicine and as a ritual artefact: it was used as an offering to the goddess Hecate, and was invoked as a deity by the Egyptians of this period during the swearing of oaths. Later, in the time of the Roman Empire, it was transported throughout Europe by soldiers and their doctors: they would plant it wherever they travelled, to use as food and medicine. They knew it would help them fight off ear, nose, throat and chest infections, and help keep their wounds clean.

The Roman writer Pliny and the physician Galen both held garlic in high regard for its medicinal properties, but not everyone appreciated its virtues. The poet Horace considered that to smell of it was vulgar. He called it 'more poisonous than hemlock' (this is completely erroneous) and wrote that he was once made ill by eating it at the table of a friend (possible, if he had a delicate digestive system). There was also a Roman superstition that garlic could destroy the magnetic properties of lodestone, a naturally-occurring magnetic material used to make an early compass—they obviously thought of it as potent stuff.

In Britain, accounts of its use date back to Saxon times. Its common name is derived from the Saxon words *gar* (a spear) and *lac* (a plant), a reference to the long, narrow shape of the leaves. In later times it was often a cause of controversy, both among ordinary people with their conflicting folklore and superstitions (most people have heard of its Gothic reputation as a vampire repellent), and among doctors who held strong opinions either for or against it. The famous apothecary and herbalist Nicholas Culpeper (1616–1664) was a great advocate of it, for 'it helpeth the biting of mad-dogs and other venomous creatures; it killeth worms in children, cutteth and bringeth forth tough phlegm, purgeth the head, helpeth the lethargy, and is a good preservative against, and a remedy for, any plague-sore or foul ulcer.' However, his predecessor John Gerard (1545–1607), master-surgeon and writer of an equally prestigious herbal, was much more sceptical about its properties.

Throughout the seventeenth and eighteenth centuries there was the hope that an effective treatment for the devastating epidemic diseases would be found, and the use of garlic was popular against leprosy, smallpox, the plague and tuberculosis. There were numerous folk recipes for preparations containing garlic, in syrups and vinegars, to be used for chest infections and asthma.

Herbalists have traditionally considered garlic to be a 'warming' remedy. The division of herbal remedies into classes of 'warming' and 'cooling' is very different from the approach of orthodox medicine, but is a most useful consideration for natural practitioners. Most people, if asked, would know whether or not they usually feel warm, or if they have a tendency to feel the cold severely. This can be related broadly to the efficiency of their circulation. When formulating a combination of remedies, if a herbalist is treating a warm-constitution person, the choice of at least some of them will be different from those chosen for someone with a cold constitution. As garlic has so many benefits for the circulation, it is not surprising that it is classed as a warming remedy. Many herbalists refer to it as a remedy that will promote sweating, another function associated with becoming warm.

During the First World War the treatment of soldiers' wounds was a doctor's nightmare: in the poor conditions of the field hospitals it was impossible to prevent them becoming infected. In 1916 the British government made an appeal for garlic to use as an antiseptic, offering one shilling per pound weight of it. The fresh juice was pressed out, diluted with water and added to dressings of sterilised sphagnum moss which were then applied to the wounds. Reports of the results suggest that thousands of soldiers were saved from amputations or death with this treatment.

Towards the end of the Second World War, garlic's antibiotic constituents and their precursor substances were isolated by an American chemical company. The puzzle of why whole raw garlic has virtually no smell whereas crushed garlic does, and why this is lost again when the garlic is cooked at high temperatures, was at last solved. It was revealed that whole raw garlic possesses an odourless sulphur-containing substance called *alliin*. When the clove is crushed this is brought into contact with an enzyme (a substance that promotes biological reactions but itself remains unchanged by the processes) called *allinase*. This changes the alliin to the characteristically pungent-smelling *allicin*, the rather acrid substance that can cause the sense of irritation when raw garlic is eaten. Allicin is the source of further active constituents. It breaks down spontaneously, over a fairly short period of time, into other sulphur-containing substances that produce the final range of therapeutic actions. So there is a chain of constituents and chemical changes between the whole raw clove and the final active remedy. The reason why highly-cooked garlic loses its pungency is that extreme heat will destroy allicin. There is then no starter substance from which the final range of active constituents can be formed.

Since these discoveries in 1944, thousands of studies have been carried out. They have confirmed the use of garlic, as the whole clove or in tablet form, as an antibiotic. It works against a wide range of bacteria, viruses, protozoa (single-celled organisms) and parasites. In the past, when the scourges of life were the virulent, life-threatening infections, these were the properties that were recognised and valued. In many developing parts of the world its anti-infective properties are still its most useful characteristic. Even nowadays, in the developed countries, many people still take it for some extra protection against the risk of respiratory and digestive tract infections. But there is another benefit that has become apparent and much more relevant to the late twentieth-century epidemic of heart disease: many recent studies have concerned the protective effect against high blood cholesterol levels and the risk of thrombosis. This raises garlic to the status of one of the most universally valuable herbal remedies known.

Garlic has other benefits that deserve recognition. It is useful in stimulating the digestive processes, including the production of bile by the liver. Bile has two roles: it helps to excrete certain unwanted substances, including cholesterol (which will add to the total cholesterol-lowering action) and bile acids. These then play a role in the breakdown of fats in the digestive tract, and add to the efficiency of fat absorption. A good supply of bile helps to reduce the risk of constipation, by easing the passage of the stool through the gut. Garlic also helps to stimulate the production of insulin by the pancreas. Insulin is responsible for keeping the level of sugar in the blood within its healthy range: diabetics do not make enough of it to achieve this. Garlic is therefore a useful addition to the diet of people who have a tendency to produce too little insulin, if they are in the group who have been recommended by their doctor to control their blood sugar by dietary means. **Caution: garlic is *not* an alternative to orthodox medication for diabetes.**

Garlic is a species within the class of plants called *angiosperms* (meaning that the seeds are formed within a protective structure) which represents most of the flowering plants we see today. The origin of the angiosperms is uncertain, but they first appeared in the Early Cretaceous period, about 60 million years ago, well after the dinosaurs became extinct. As garlic is a member of the order Liliflorae, it is a distant relative of the amaryllis and iris, and as a member of the Liliaceae family it is a closer relative of the lily of the valley (*Convallaria majalis*) and Solomon's seal (*Polygonatum multiflorum*) among others. Within the genus *Allium* are its closest relatives, the onion (*Allium cepa*) and the wild garlic or ramsons

Figure 1 The place of *Allium sativum* within the plant kingdom*

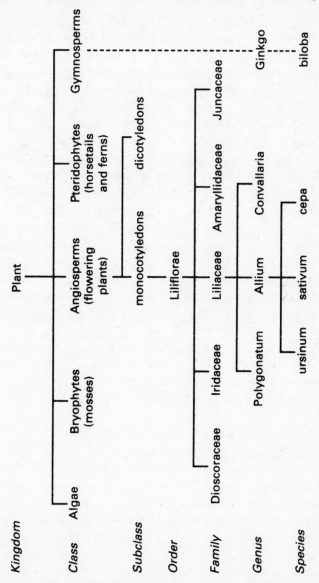

*Note: many plants and groups have been omitted for the sake of clarity

(*Allium ursinum*). These relationships are summarised in Figure 1.

Although we do not know when garlic evolved as a species, we know that the group of plants to which it belongs started to develop about 50 million years ago. Ginkgo, in contrast, has a history that goes back to and even predates the dinosaurs. Fossil ginkgos over 250 million years old have been found. They proliferated in the Permian period (from 285 to 250 million years ago), replacing the giant club mosses and horsetails of the Carboniferous period. They developed at the same time as conifers, seed ferns, gnetales and cycads, and recent research has suggested that of this ancient group ginkgo and gnetales are the oldest (Chaw *et al*). Of the many species of ancient ginkgo, only one remains, *Ginkgo biloba*, earning for itself the title of 'living fossil'. This became restricted to China and may well have become extinct in the wild a few thousand years ago, surviving only through the efforts of the Chinese population to conserve it for its economic value as a source of food, timber and medicine. In the tenth century it was actively planted in Kaifeng, the capital city of the Sung dynasty, and by the seventeenth century had been taken to Japan. Buddhist monks favoured the beauty of ginkgo trees and planted them extensively around their temples. European travellers brought them from the East in the eighteenth century, and ginkgo is now widely cultivated in North America and Europe. Large plantations have been established in France and America and the annual sales of ginkgo-based products in Europe now amount to more than £100 million.

The seeds have economic value: they are rich in oils that have been used in soap-making (but they also smell very unpleasant after a few days and can give rise to an allergic skin reaction, so must be handled cautiously). The inner nut is something of a forbidden fruit: it has a pleasant, sweet taste, but contains toxic constituents. In the East it is regarded as a delicacy, but it has to be carefully prepared and cooked. Even then, the amount that can be safely eaten is small, so my advice is to avoid it completely.

In the system of botanical classification, ginkgo is an extremely distant relative of garlic, being a gymnosperm (meaning 'naked

Figure 2   The place of *Ginkgo biloba* within the plant kingdom*

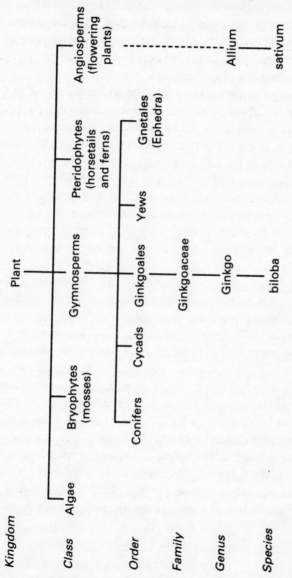

*Note: many plants and groups have been omitted for the sake of clarity

seed', as the seed develops without any surrounding protective structure), an ancient division of the plant kingdom which includes conifers, yews and cycads, gnetales and the ginkgoales. Within the order of Ginkgoales comes the family Ginkgoaceae of which *Ginkgo biloba* is the only member. Figure 2 outlines the place of ginkgo within the plant kingdom.

Like garlic in the Middle East, ginkgo has been used in Chinese medicine for about 5,000 years. Written accounts of its specific use date back to 2800 BC and it appeared regularly in later medical treatises. In the most famous, the *Pen Ts'ao Kan Mu*, written by Li Shih-Chen in the late sixteenth century, there is a written entry and an illustration of the foliage and fruit. It was classed with those remedies indicated for 'expelling phlegm', and is still an ingredient in a classical combination to relieve chest problems. In modern China, where herbal medicine is accepted and used alongside more recently developed drug treatments, it is used for cardiovascular and chest problems.

In the West, ginkgo does not have the traditional reputation of garlic and has only recently started to appear in the medical literature and herbals. It was the growing interest in alternative medicine and traditional Chinese remedies that brought ginkgo to the attention of Western medical practitioners, and within the last ten years there has been considerable research into its biochemical composition. Ginkgo has some extremely complex chemicals, the structure of which has only recently been determined. The plant has been found to contain a wide range of active components from the three main classes of chemicals found in plants, *nitrogen compounds* (predominantly alkaloids), *terpenoids* and *phenolics*. As we shall see in the following chapters, these constituents are extremely useful in treating a diverse range of disorders, including cardiovascular problems, psoriasis, ischaemia and pre-menstrual tension.

CHAPTER 2

How Your Heart and Circulation Work

Before discussing the treatment of cardiovascular problems with garlic and ginkgo, we need to know a little about what the cardiovascular system does and how it works. We also need to look at the causes of various common disorders of the system and what happens when it goes wrong.

Few families in the Western world can have remained unaffected by the epidemic of diseases of the heart and blood vessels: current figures show that each year, in the UK alone, more than 180,000 people die from heart attacks, thrombosis, embolism or strokes, and many more are left permanently disabled. In 1990 the cost to the National Health Service for the care and treatment of this type of heart disease was well over 50 million pounds. Diseases with a similar cause include angina pectoris, intermittent claudication and senility due to an inadequate supply of blood to the brain, and some types of hypertension (high blood pressure). There is one pathological problem underlying all these different manifestations of disease: deterioration of the condition of the arteries with the build-up of blockages to the blood-flow.

THE CIRCULATORY SYSTEM

Blood is the fluid of life, it is necessary to every cell in our body and no cell is more than one millimetre distant from a blood vessel. It delivers vital nutrients and oxygen, which enable our cells to produce energy and the materials they need to function. It removes waste products such as carbon dioxide and urea which become toxic if they accumulate. It provides a communication system, transporting chemical messenger molecules called hormones from the glands in which they are produced to the target organs and tissues where they initiate a change in function. It plays a role in our defences against harmful micro-organisms, by carrying white cells that fight off the 'invaders'.

The circulatory system, comprising the heart, blood vessels and blood, can be thought of as the body's internal transport system, bearing messages and materials from one part of the body to another. The system is also central to the maintenance of the internal balance of physical functions, known as *homoeostasis*. It is closely integrated with the processes that control nutrient levels and waste disposal, as well as water and temperature regulation.

The need for an internal transport system arose many millions of years ago, when an increase in the size and complexity of multicellular animals became limited by the rate at which gases and nutrients could be obtained from the external environment by simple *diffusion* (the tendency of small molecules to move through the membranes into the interior of the cells). The development of a simple circulation meant that exchange could be managed by specialist organs such as the gut and lungs and the products of exchange transported to all the cells of the body. It would be reasonable to suggest that without the development of the circulatory system, animal life as we know it today would not exist.

At the centre of the system is the heart, a large, muscular pump which beats seventy or so times each minute from a few weeks after conception to the last minutes of the individual's life. A simple calculation indicates that, by the age of seventy, the heart has beaten over 2.5 billion times. The heart is not a single pump but two separate pumps joined together and beating in unison. The right side sends blood to the lungs, from where it returns to the left side of the heart. From here the blood is sent around the capillaries which supply blood to the tissues and organs of the body (the *systemic circulation*). The blood then returns to the right side from where it is again sent around the lungs. A simplified diagram of the circulatory system is shown in Figure 3.

One of the most important functions of the circulatory system is the transport of gases to and from the tissues and the lungs. In the lungs blood receives oxygen from the air and gets rid of the waste gas carbon dioxide. In the systemic circulation, oxygen is delivered to the tissues from the blood which then collects the carbon dioxide and transports it back to the lungs for disposal. An overview of the exchange of gases in the circulatory system is shown in Figure 4.

The network of blood vessels that conducts blood to and from all parts of the body is called the vascular system. The vessels in various parts of the system are different in structure to make them suited to their particular function. Those conducting blood from the heart to the tissues are called *arteries*. They vary in size from 2.5 centimetres for the aorta, down to 30 micrometres (three thousandths of a centimetre) for the small arterioles. They have a lot of muscle fibres and elastic fibres in their walls, so that they can both stretch and constrict to alter their diameter when required. This alternate stretching and recoil creates the force that pushes the blood continuously through the vessels (rather than only when the heart is in the pumping phase of its cycle).

The arteries branch into smaller muscular-walled vessels, which in turn branch into *capillaries*. These are only five thousandths of a millimetre in diameter and their walls are just one cell thick, being the same type of cells that form the lining of the larger blood vessels. It is in the capillaries that the exchange of materials between the blood and the tissues takes place, and although they are so small, they form a total area for exchange of 6,300 square metres throughout the body. The capillaries then join to form larger vessels, which in turn form the larger *veins*. These return the blood to the heart. Their walls are thinner than those of the arteries, but they do have a certain amount of muscle fibre, and the larger veins have some elastic fibres as well. They can alter their diameter to vary the amount of blood they hold, which controls the amount of blood returned to the heart. Veins have one-way valves at

Figure 3   Schematic diagram of the circulatory system

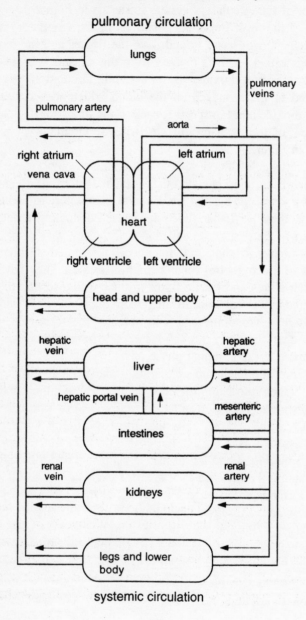

pulmonary circulation

lungs

pulmonary veins

pulmonary artery

aorta

right atrium

left atrium

vena cava

heart

right ventricle   left ventricle

head and upper body

hepatic vein

hepatic artery

liver

hepatic portal vein

mesenteric artery

intestines

renal vein

renal artery

kidneys

legs and lower body

systemic circulation

Figure 4   Gas exchange in the circulatory system

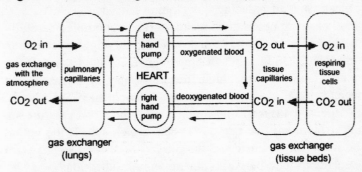

The capillary networks in the body tissues and lungs act as gas exchangers. Oxygen (O_2) diffuses into the blood capillaries from the air in the lungs and is carried around the body by the circulatory system. In the body tissues, the oxygen diffuses out of the blood capillaries into the tissue cells and is replaced by carbon dioxide (CO_2) which is transported in the blood to the lungs. Here it diffuses out of the blood capillaries into the air in the lungs and is replaced by oxygen.

intervals along their length, to prevent the back-flow of blood from the lower part of the body as it returns upwards towards the heart.

Blood that has received oxygen as it passed through the lungs (and is bright red as a result) is carried from the heart under high pressure through the arteries. You can feel the stretch and recoil this pressure causes as the pulse at your wrist from the *radial artery*, and at various other places in the body where an artery is close to the surface of the skin, such as the *carotid pulse* in the neck (very important for checking that blood is getting through to the brain). Blood that has given up its oxygen in the capillaries (and is dark-coloured) is returned to the heart, under less pressure, through the veins.

The blood pressure is determined by the rate and strength of the heart contraction, the tension in the walls of the smaller arteries (called *arterioles*) and the viscosity or 'stickiness' of the blood itself. This stickiness is due to a type of blood cell called a *platelet*. There are about 200,000 to 400,000 platelets in each cubic millimetre of blood. They function to prevent excess leakage of blood from any damaged vessel by starting the blood-clotting mechanism into action. When people refer to the need to keep the blood 'thin' they mean ways of reducing this clotting tendency.

Blood pressure needs to be maintained and controlled carefully by the body. If it is too low to overcome the high resistance in the arterioles, then insufficient blood may reach the tissues. If, on the other hand, it is too high, the heart may be stressed, and damage, especially rupture of the small peripheral blood vessels, may ensue. The mechanisms which control the blood pressure are complex, involving the nervous system which adjusts the output of the heart and diameter of the blood vessels and longer-term adjustments of total blood volume, mainly by the kidneys.

DISORDERS OF THE CIRCULATORY SYSTEM

As we get older it seems that most of us develop signs of certain problems with the health of our blood vessels. These have probably started years previously, in early life, with the deposition of fatty material on the linings of the blood vessels. The deposits are made from *cholesterol* and other fats (also known as lipids), and are termed *atheromatous plaques*. They become larger and more numerous as we get older, and in severe cases they can block up to three-quarters of the diameter of the vessel. This obviously greatly reduces the flow of blood through the affected vessel. The wall surrounding the plaques can be invaded by cells that form scar-like tissue, which then attracts the deposition of the mineral calcium. The vessel then becomes hardened and inelastic, which causes functional problems, particularly in the arteries. This is known as *arteriosclerosis*.

The force of the pulse wave is absorbed by the elasticity in the arteries, and when this is lost there is likely to be an increase in blood pressure during the pumping phase of the heart's contraction/relaxation cycle. People are generally not aware of these problems developing until the plaques have become so large that they impede the normal flow of blood to the tissues served by the particular artery, at which stage the condition is called *atherosclerosis*.

The problem will be noticed more quickly if the affected tissues are those that need a plentiful supply of blood to meet the demands of the work they do. For instance, during exercise the heart itself has to work harder, so it will need an increased supply of blood to meet its own requirement for extra oxygen. Atheromas in the heart's own arteries can leave the heart muscle without an adequate supply of oxygen, and as the tissues struggle to produce energy this may cause the pain known as *angina pectoris* (a fuller description of this condition is given on p. 32). A similar problem can affect a person's calf muscles if the arteries to the legs are affected by atheroma in a disease referred to as *intermittent claudication* (the Roman emperor Claudius suffered from this). Again, a cramp-like pain comes on during walking, and forces the sufferer to stand still until it subsides.

In the brain, a reduction of blood supply can cause periods of confusion and poor memory called *transient ischaemia*. This may be difficult to distinguish from actual deterioration of the nerve cells themselves (such as in Alzheimer's disease), as the symptoms are very similar. However, when the problem is caused by a temporary reduction in blood supply to the brain, the symptoms usually improve when it returns to normal.

Thrombosis in the arteries

The formation of an atherosclerotic plaque on the lining of an artery can also lead to the formation of a blood clot or *thrombus*, and if the blood clot breaks free of its attachment it becomes an *embolus* (a name given to any extraneous object transported in the blood) and can travel in the circulation until it becomes lodged in a smaller blood vessel, causing a *thromboembolism*. If this vessel is in the heart or brain, areas of tissue may be deprived of blood and the results may be very serious indeed. The formation of a thrombus is quite complex, but an understanding of the process can help us appreciate the action of the various remedies discussed in this book and also the importance of the preventative measures we can take to keep our circulatory system healthy. This process is described more fully in chapter 9.

Coronary heart disease

Circulatory problems directly affecting the supply of blood to the heart itself are called *coronary heart disease*. The heart has its own blood supply via the coronary arteries which branch off the aorta and form an inverted crown-shaped web of arteries (hence the name 'coronary'). A severe reduction in the flow of blood to the heart causes an area of heart muscle to be deprived of oxygen and nutrients and is then said to be *ischaemic*. If the blood supply is withheld for more than one hour the cells of the heart muscle may die and the area of dead cells is called an *infarction*. The extent of the affected area depends on the point at which the blockage occurs and whether blood from adjacent arteries can take over the supply of blood from the blocked arteries (see Figure 5). A blockage in a large artery will obviously deprive a large area of muscle of its blood and thus be potentially more serious than a blockage in one of the smaller arteries. Atherosclerosis, the build-up of fatty plaques, may cause a progressive narrowing of the arteries. The coronary arteries which supply blood to the heart muscle are susceptible to atheroma, particularly the left coronary artery. As the blockage of the arteries increases, the flow of blood with its supply of oxygen for the heart muscle decreases. The muscle cells of the heart do not get enough oxygen and this causes the cells to produce *lactic acid*. As the heart responds very quickly to quite small increases in physical activity, such as walking and climbing stairs, this increase in the heart rate results in a rapid increase in lactic acid production, causing the pain known as *angina pectoris*. Angina is often the first sign of atheroma in the coronary arteries.

This condition may lead to the formation of a thrombus, a clumping of platelets and blood cells in a fibrous mesh—otherwise known as a clot. If this breaks free it will move with the blood flow along increasingly narrowing blood vessels until it gets stuck, completely blocking the vessel and becoming a *thromboembolism*. This will deprive an area of tissue of its blood supply as described above.

When this happens, the normal electrical activity of the heart

Figure 5   The effect of thrombosis on the coronary arteries

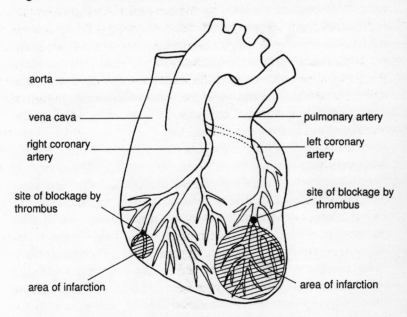

The area of heart muscle affected depends largely on the site of occlusion. The larger the artery which is blocked by a thrombus, the larger will be the area deprived of blood. The above diagram shows two possible sites of blockage and the resulting differences in the size of infarctions.

which controls the smooth and regular contraction of the heart muscle may be disrupted, causing erratic beating called *arrhythmias*. Serious arrhythmias may lead to *ventricular fibrillation*, uncoordinated and weak contractions of the chambers of the heart, causing a reduction in blood pressure and even death in extreme circumstances.

Preventative treatment of individuals susceptible to coronary heart disease is usually by drugs which reduce the 'stickiness' of the blood or prevent platelet clumping. Surgery in severe cases may involve grafting a blood vessel, usually a vein from the leg, from the aorta to a point on the coronary artery beyond the blockage. Sometimes two or more grafts need to be done, hence double and triple bypass operations. An alternative approach, which does not involve opening the chest cavity, is called *percutaneous transluminal coronary angioplasty* (PTCA for short). Using special imaging techniques, a catheter is carefully guided along an artery from the patient's arm or leg to the site of blockage in the coronary artery. A balloon on the end of the catheter is then inflated, which squashes the atheroma and widens the artery. To prevent the artery closing up again, a plastic coil called a stent may be left in the repaired artery to maintain blood flow.

Deep vein thrombosis

Clots which form in the deep veins of the legs are often unassociated with atheroma or damaged blood vessels and the cause of their formation is not fully understood. It is possible that platelet clumping may begin at one of the small valves found in the veins, but most certainly the condition is aggravated by poor blood flow. Those most at risk are patients undergoing surgery or suffering from cancer, but obesity has also been implicated, as well as the use of steroid hormones such as oestrogen.

A deep vein thrombus of the leg breaking loose from the vein and forming a travelling blood clot, now called an embolus, may well be expected to produce a different result from arterial thromboembolism. In the case of deep vein thrombosis, the clot is travelling into wider and wider veins rather than, in the case of the arteries, where the blood flows from larger to smaller blood vessels. The deep vein thrombus is most likely to travel to the right side of the heart. From the heart its destination is almost certainly the lungs where the blockage of a pulmonary artery will result in a *pulmonary embolism*. This may place such a strain on the heart as it struggles to pump against this sudden increase in arterial pressure that *acute heart failure* can be caused.

High blood pressure (hypertension)

Blood pressure is measured by a device called a *sphygmomanometer* which used to involve wrapping a cuff around the upper arm and pumping a column of mercury up and down a scale whilst the doctor listened to arterial sounds at the inner elbow with a stethoscope. These days, digital equipment is used, which takes the measurements automatically and displays the results on a digital readout. Usually two figures are given, typically 120/80 mmHg. The higher figure represents the pressure when the heart has contracted and forced blood into the arteries, and the lower figure is the pressure when the heart is relaxed and arterial pressure falls. High blood pressure or *hypertension* is defined as being consistently above 140/90 mmHg.

The cause of high blood pressure is often difficult to establish and in 90 per cent of cases it remains unknown. In those cases where the cause can be established it is usually the result of another disorder, such as kidney disease or hormone imbalances—in other words, it is secondary to that disorder. Cardiovascular hypertension caused by atherosclerotic plaques partially blocking the arteries is a common cause of high blood pressure. Unfortunately, atherosclerosis is also an effect of hypertension and it has been shown that plaques are formed more readily when blood pressure is high. Put another way, atherosclerosis causes hypertension which promotes atherosclerosis . . . and so on.

Hypertension is associated with smoking, obesity, stress and a high salt diet. It may also run in families. Treatment may mean a change in lifestyle such as giving up smoking and a different diet, along with treatment with anti-hypertensive drugs. These are divided into two groups. *Diuretics* increase the amount of water extracted from the blood by the kidneys and lost in urine. This has the effect of lowering the total blood volume and thus blood pressure. The second group are drugs specific to hypertension, such as *beta blockers* which keep the heart rate down, and *calcium antagonists* which open up the smaller arteries.

CHAPTER 3

Make the Most of Your Brain

The most popular use for ginkgo in Europe is in the treatment of *cerebral insufficiency* (lack of adequate blood supply to the brain). How, then, does the brain function in health and illness?

Of all the organs in the human body, the brain is the most complex in structure and also the least well understood in its functioning. It is the main control centre of the body, responsible for receiving information from the senses of touch, taste, sight, hearing and smell, processing that information and then sending instructions to the organs and muscles of the body, as well as allowing us to understand what is happening. If you want to imagine how complex a job the brain can do, think of a concert pianist playing a really fast Liszt piano concerto. The eyes read the notes off the music score and send signals to the brain which translates the notes on the page into signals to the fingers about which keys to strike and when to strike them. At the same time the pianist is listening to the music and thinking about interpretation, and whilst all of this is going on the brain is also controlling the pianist's breathing, digestion and many other automatic body functions.

With such a complex organ it is obviously important that it is kept healthy and working properly. In normal life, exercise, a good diet and plenty of sleep should be sufficient to ensure that the brain continues to do its job efficiently. As we get older, our bodies start to show signs of age and sometimes of neglect, and in the case of the brain this can lead to various disorders that may prevent us from enjoying life to the full. However, with a sensible lifestyle, and with the help of such herbs as ginkgo and garlic, it is possible to give our brains and other organs the best chance of a long and healthy life.

All the nerves throughout the body, and the brain itself, are composed of the same types of tissue. There are two kinds of cells: those that do the prime work of communication and the others that play a protective and supportive role to help them achieve this. The communication is achieved by the transmission of tiny electrical impulses over the surface membrane of cells called *neurons*. Special chemicals called *neurotransmitters* carry the impulse from one neuron to the next, bridging the minute gap between them. Nerves are composed of the long fibres of neurons in bundles that lead from all parts of the body, enter the spinal cord and then connect with neurons in the brain. The electrical impulses thus travel along the nerve fibres, providing a pathway for communication from the body to the brain. Other nerves contain neurons that transmit impulses out from the brain and down to all parts of the body.

The neurons in the brain itself are very similar to those in the nerves, but they have shorter fibres and far more connections to other neurons, and they form extremely complex networks for the transmission of impulses. Some areas of the brain are stimulated by the incoming nerve impulses, resulting in the various physical sensations we experience. Other areas initiate the impulses that are transmitted back to the body, resulting in changes of function such as movement, shivering or sweating, changes in heart-rate, blood pressure and so on. Thus damage in particular areas of the brain can cause the loss of either sensory functions or the ability to perform certain actions, depending on where the damage occurs.

Human beings have evolved larger brains than most other animals, with areas of spare capacity that are not needed for sensing or controlling our bodies. These are called *association areas*, and they allow the neural network to make complex connections between different parts of the brain. These extra connections, which most animal brains don't have room for, create our numerous abstract intellectual abilities such as rational patterns of thought, planning ahead, inventiveness and so on. These enable us to live all over the earth, in the most inhospitable climates, by allowing us to develop the social relationships and invent the technology that help us to survive.

The brain needs a rich supply of oxygen and glucose as sources of energy to carry out its work. Unlike many other tissues, brain can use only glucose, not fats, to provide its energy needs. An indication of how important the brain is in the hierarchy of the body organs is that it is the only organ that does not need the hormone insulin to help it absorb glucose. When there is plenty of glucose available in the blood, insulin is produced so that all tissues can absorb it. But when blood sugar levels drop, insulin production ceases temporarily and only the brain is still able to absorb glucose, giving it 'preferential treatment' to enable it to carry on its vital functions.

The brain receives about 15 per cent of the total output of blood from the heart. It consumes about 18 per cent of the body's total oxygen content, with only the liver and skeletal muscles (and these only during physical exercise) requiring more. Brain cells need a constant supply of oxygen and glucose, and are particularly susceptible to damage if the supply is interrupted. There is also a protective system of membranes and cells called the *blood-brain barrier* that prevents the passage of any harmful substances from the bloodstream into the brain tissues. The supply of blood necessary to keep the brain working properly is provided by four arteries which form a ring under its base. Thus if there is an interruption in the supply from one of the arteries, it can be compensated for by the supply from the others.

It will be obvious that any condition of the blood vessels that restricts the flow of blood to the brain will have serious consequences. *Cerebral insufficiency* occurs when the blood supply is reduced but not completely blocked, causing a gradual impairment of mental faculties. As people get older it is expected that some faculties, such as memory, reasoning ability and concentration, will diminish. This deterioration will vary between individuals, and some people who survive into their nineties remain bright and alert. The causes of mental impairment are complex, difficult to diagnose and often due to other disorders such as infections and metabolic imbalances. When correctly treated, there can be a resulting improvement in mental as well as physical symptoms. However, any degree of cerebral insufficiency is likely to aggravate other causes of mental impairment. Given the commonness of circulatory deterioration among elderly people nowadays, it is likely that some component of mental impairment will be due to cerebral insufficiency and its consequences. Where this is diagnosed, treatment may involve surgery, or drugs which will keep the blood thin and improve its flow through the partly blocked arteries.

Strokes, in contrast, are caused by a sudden loss of blood to an area of brain tissue. The extent of the damage will depend on the site of the blockage and the ability of other arteries to supply blood to the affected area. The two major causes of strokes are atherosclerosis in one of the arteries carrying blood to the brain and high blood pressure. In the case of atherosclerosis, this is most common in the carotid arteries. One of the first signs of stroke may be *transient ischaemic attacks* (TIA), literally, a short-term disorder caused by an interruption in the blood supply to a particular area of tissue. TIAs usually last for only a few minutes and symptoms may include interference with vision, vertigo, confusion, slurred speech or falling to the ground (without loss of consciousness). The frequency of the attacks may vary depending on the cause of the problem, but in some cases sufferers may experience several attacks in one day or they may occur only once or twice a year. Treatment may involve surgery to repair the damaged arteries, but more usually, as with cerebral insufficiency, drugs are prescribed to keep the blood thin and flowing well.

TIAs caused by high blood pressure will be treated with drugs appropriate to the cause of this.

If left untreated, TIAs caused by thrombosis may progress to the point where permanent damage is caused to an area of tissue which has been deprived of blood and the cells may die from lack of oxygen and nutrients. If a clot breaks free from an atheromatous plaque it can cause a *complete stroke*. In this case damage to the brain, and the symptoms caused by the damage, may be permanent. If the blood supply returns (called *reperfusion*) before cell death occurs, other damage may still be caused as the returning blood itself triggers the production of a substance called *platelet activating factor*. This leads to swelling of the brain and the formation of substances that are toxic to the neurons. Further problems are caused by the formation of highly damaging *free radicals* (see p. 53). These changes cause an escalation of the damage due to the original deprivation of blood. So it can be appreciated that any remedies able to limit the extent of the damage have a valuable role to play in the treatment of cerebrovascular diseases.

CHAPTER 4

Asthma—Breathing Made Difficult

Remarkable though it may seem, ginkgo and garlic are as useful in the treatment of asthma as they are with cardiovascular problems. To understand this, we need to look more closely at what the term 'asthma' means.

Most people are familiar with the unpleasant sensation of 'tightness' in the chest that is a common symptom of chest infections. It feels as if the airways, the tubes leading into the lungs, won't open up enough to allow the lungs to fill comfortably with air, and this is actually what happens. These tubes (the larger ones are called *bronchi*, the smaller ones *bronchioles*) have rings of muscle along their length. When these muscles contract they narrow the diameter of the bronchi, which makes the flow of air along them much more restricted. The problem is compounded because this reaction is usually caused by irritation or damage to the mucous membranes lining the airways. This will provoke swelling of the membranes along with the production of mucus as a protective mechanism. The mucus is often very thick and jelly-like, and difficult to cough up. So the air passages are further narrowed, restricting the amount of air able to get through.

The consequence is that not enough oxygen gets through to the lungs, and therefore not enough enters the blood as it passes through the lungs. If the membranes remain swollen and inflamed over a period of time they become infiltrated by immune cells. Bacteria invade the mucus, making the chances of infection more likely, and damage to the membranes prevents them from carrying

41

out their normal cleansing functions of wafting the mucus upwards and out of the lungs. There is a characteristic wheezy sound to the breathing of a person suffering from asthma. The amount of effort being put into the breathing will be obvious, and the discomfort and anxiety it causes can be very distressing.

There are varying degrees of severity to the problem, ranging from a mild discomfort and perhaps a dry cough, to a sudden and severe difficulty with breathing. The duration of the disturbance to breathing is also very variable—it could be either a short attack with the person feeling quite well at other times, or it could be prolonged and even a semi-permanent state. It can be brought on by different causes, or may be an inherited tendency. The basic mechanism seems to be an allergic response, but this can be aggravated by other factors such as a chest infection, excitement or stress, and smoke or other air pollutants. The substances provoking the allergy may be in the environment, such as the pollen that also causes hay fever symptoms, or the microscopic droppings from house mites, or in some cases may be foods that go unsuspected because they are a usual item of the diet. Cow's milk and its derivatives are sometimes responsible, and an allergic person's symptoms may be much reduced simply by cutting out all foods that contain these. Some people develop asthma after having repeated chest infections or bronchitis, and constriction of the airways can complicate other lung diseases such as emphysema.

The mechanism that causes the constriction and swelling in the air passages is complex and not fully understood. It is thought to involve the interaction of various types of cell, notably the platelets in the blood, and also other cells from the lining of the air passages and those of the immune system. The end result is some degree of obstruction to breathing.

Asthma is not a new disease and evidence of its existence goes back at least 7,000 years. It seems that nowadays, however, the incidence of asthma, especially among the young of the developed, industrialised nations, is on the increase. Over ten per cent of children in the UK are affected with asthma and between five and ten per cent of adults. The problem with quantifying changes in the prevalence of the condition is in defining it, as it is very difficult to collect asthmatics into one clearly identifiable group. A common working definition of asthma is *reversible bronchial airflow obstruction*, but this may cover a wide range of patients with symptoms ranging from occasional wheezing to acute severe asthma (which can in some cases be fatal). Definitions apart, most medical practitioners will have little problem recognising the majority of cases they see.

Asthma can be divided broadly into two categories, *intrinsic* and *extrinsic*. Most cases of childhood asthma are extrinsic, attacks being induced by specific trigger substances. With appropriate treatment the disease is often reversible and may disappear completely in time. Adult onset asthma falls more frequently into the intrinsic category and its causes may be infections, often viral, leading to chronic and only partially reversible bronchial obstruction.

Common triggers of asthma include house mites, pollen, pet fur, house dust, cold air and exercise. Identification of the factor concerned can be very helpful in reducing the severity of the symptoms (although some triggers such as house mites and house dust are so pervasive that it is almost impossible to create an environment free from them). Some asthmas may arise from a person's type of occupation, recognisable by an improvement in symptoms during weekends and holidays.

There has been controversy as to whether an increase in air pollution, specifically that produced by road traffic, is a major factor in the increasing incidence of childhood asthma. Certainly, during periods of severe atmospheric pollution and smogs, more people are admitted to hospital suffering from asthma, but against this is the fact that there is generally very little difference in the frequency of asthma between rural and urban areas. The picture of cause and effect is not clear and studies have failed to show any firm connection.

A recent study in Germany looked at the question of air pollution and asthma and also at childhood exposure to potential *allergens* (substances that can trigger allergic reactions in susceptible people). The researchers looked at the frequency of childhood asthma in Germany before reunification. In West Germany, which was relatively affluent, pollution levels were low and the percentage of children diagnosed as asthmatic was high, whereas in the poorer and more heavily polluted East Germany (GDR) there were relatively few cases of asthma. Contrasting with this, respiratory infections were low in West Germany whilst in East Germany there was a high rate of bronchitis and other respiratory infections.

The study suggested that air pollution was not the prime cause of childhood asthma in West Germany, the main factor being the prevalence of centrally heated houses and fitted carpets, ideal conditions for dust mites (one of the most common triggers of extrinsic asthma). It also suggested that exposure to infections, plus the lack of fitted carpets and central heating in East Germany, conferred some protection against asthma. This latter finding has been backed by other research: it is thought that in developed countries, where well-organised immunisation programmes, together with readily available antibiotics, reduce the number of childhood infections, the child's immune system may not be challenged sufficiently to mature properly. This somehow causes the unused capacity of the immune system to switch from recognising infections to a sensitisation to other common substances such as dust mites and pollen.

It must be emphasised here that parents should not be deterred from having their children immunised against those childhood diseases, such as diphtheria and polio, which have in past generations claimed many young lives. However, it does throw doubt on the value of using antibiotics against minor childhood infections: this practice may well prove to be a causative factor in the increasing incidence of childhood asthma.

CHAPTER 5

What You Can Do to Stay Healthy

What are the reasons for the epidemic of cardiovascular disease? As more research is done it all points to one broad cause—that our way of life is changing rapidly towards an increasingly sedentary state, in which we eat too much highly-processed and over-rich food. This is leading us away from the way of life that keeps us healthy, so that we end up paying a high price for our affluence.

For more than a hundred thousand years after the human race evolved, our way of life and type of food stayed the same. We ate animals caught by hunters, and leaves, fruit, nuts, seeds and roots obtained by gatherers. We might think of this as a very poor way of life compared to ours in the present, but in fact the resulting diet, so long as there was enough of it, was very varied and nourishing. Small quantities of many different foods seem to have suited us best then, and still do now. There would have been ample protein from the meat, seeds and nuts, along with small amounts of fat (wild animals have much less fat than farm-raised animals), starches from the roots and sugars from the fruits (a seasonal treat rather than year-round, of course), an adequate range of vitamins and minerals, and plenty of fibre. It involved a lot of walking and stalking, which used up energy, but so long as the total human population was small, it was a very efficient way of obtaining food. Even today, some isolated tribal peoples still follow this way of life, whilst there are still enough plant and animal species to support it.

The problem was that this way of life was so successful that

45

humans flourished to the point where there were more and more people competing for a limited food stock. Hunters and gatherers had to go farther afield to find food and thus had to put more time and energy into an increasingly inefficient lifestyle.

Eventually humans changed from collecting wild food to producing it themselves. Agricultural systems developed and provided more reliable access to food, though the overall variety was greatly reduced. There was probably much more work involved in food production than there had been previously in hunting and gathering. The nutritional content of human diets may have started to decline from then on, as the range of foods eaten became much narrower. But it was obviously still a very successful way of feeding the population, which has continued to grow ever since.

Agricultural practices stayed about the same until comparatively recent times, but since the Industrial Revolution, around two hundred years ago, the pace of change in Europe has been accelerating. In the past fifty years there has been more change than ever before. Both the amount of physical work we do and the type of food we eat in the developed world are now radically different. Sedentary desk jobs or machine operating have replaced much of the physically intensive work of previous generations. We have cars and buses to move us around instead of having to walk or cycle; the labour has been taken out of housework by domestic machinery; shop doors open automatically and lifts and escalators remove the need to climb stairs.

All these convenient, labour-saving aids were welcomed as they freed us from the boring drudgery of life. At the same time, increasing affluence and the development of the food industry have provided us with instant food. Fifty years ago a housewife's larder would have contained little except ingredients that had to be cooked into a meal. Now, our freezers are full of ready-prepared meals that just need to be heated and eaten. There are treats like biscuits and crisps in the larder and ice cream in the fridge, ready for instant consumption. Tempting new products are constantly being advertised, all of which must be delicious to be a commercial success. How is this achieved? Often by making them high in fats or sugar, the tastes that most people immediately enjoy (and which are fairly cheap to produce). We end up with a higher proportion of fats and sugar in our diet than ever before, and our bodies don't have a healthy way of dealing with them. It isn't hard to understand, then, why recent changes have affected us so severely: our bodies are still best adapted to the food and exercise needs of ancient times. We spent a hundred and fifty thousand years in that way of life, and our bodies cannot cope healthily with the recent changes.

As the results of our lifestyle changes have become apparent, certain risk factors that seem to be most closely connected with the development of cardiovascular disease have been identified. These include: *obesity, diabetes, high blood pressure, high blood cholesterol, smoking, lack of physical exercise, a high-stress occupation or home life, and a high fat but nutrient-poor diet.* Some may be beyond our control: it is thought that certain contributory factors to obesity and high blood pressure, for instance, may be inherited rather than acquired. But that still leaves the majority of them under our own control, which is the good news. The effects of most of them are not easily separated: they are related in complex ways, and some affect others, to produce the consequences of cardiovascular disease.

The positive aspect of this is that if you manage a small improvement in one factor, you may well see improvements in others almost automatically. The thought of changing your way of life might seem daunting at first, but bear in mind that it could be the biggest favour you ever do for yourself. Here are some of the positive steps you can take.

Obesity

The number of overweight or obese people in the developed world is rising sharply. Apart from the negative self-image it can cause, obesity also brings increased risks of several diseases, including coronary heart disease, high blood pressure, osteoarthritis, gall-stones, and non-insulin-dependent diabetes. Respiratory diseases like asthma can be aggravated by the mechanical difficulty in breathing.

The part of the body where the fat is stored is important in assessing your degree of risk. If you store it mainly around the hips and thighs (the pear-shaped person) you are at less risk than if you put it on around the upper abdomen (the apple shape). Fat here is more likely to affect the work of the liver, in its processing of fats and cholesterol. Women tend to be more pear-shaped before they go through the menopause, because of the effects of the female sex hormones on their bodies, but after the menopause, when the hormone levels drop, they too often develop into the apple shape. This may account for the finding that pre-menopausal women have a lower risk of cardiovascular problems than men, whereas post-menopausal women have the same risk.

The treatment of obesity, as every would-be slimmer knows, is easy in theory but incredibly difficult in practice. What is needed is to change the balance between the amount of energy consumed in food and the amount used in physical activity: reduce the former and increase the latter. If you have patience, even a small change over a long period of time will have dramatic effects. Perhaps the easiest way is not to go on a diet that drastically reduces the amount of food you eat, but to change the types of food. Cut down on the energy-rich foods, primarily those high in fats and sugars. These are usually the snack foods and processed foods, where the fat or sugar may be hidden—take to reading the nutrition information on the label. If you get hungry between meals, eat fruit instead of snack bars. You shouldn't have to sacrifice your normal meals, providing they are not laden with roast or fried foods, or covered in rich sauces. Lean meat or fish with plenty of vegetables are no problem. You will have to find the will-power to cut out all but the occasional sweets, cakes and crisps, and you will see a quicker result if you can increase the amount of exercise you take.

Exercise
Although most children participate in games and PE at school, the division is soon made between those who are naturally athletic and successful in competition, and those who are not (and who tend to dislike it due to their feeling of low achievement). At

home, playing games out of doors has declined as homework, the TV and computers have become the more usual way of spending time. The great majority of teenagers, especially girls, stop exercising when they leave school.

These habits of inactivity, encouraged by labour-saving devices and available transport, have now become the norm for most people. Lack of exercise is connected with the problems of overweight and obesity in that, although most people now have a diet that contains fewer calories than that of previous generations, far more people are overweight because they use up less energy in physical activity.

To maintain health and wellbeing, we need to make a conscious effort to take more exercise. The benefits are proven: as we stimulate the circulation and respiratory system with the increased demands of brisk exercise, all the bodily functions involved become more efficient at meeting those demands. An improvement in cardiovascular health results after a few months. Your blood pressure can come down, your heart becomes more efficient, the blood supply to muscles is improved, breathing is easier, you can lose excess weight more quickly, strengthen your bones, look better, and feel less depressed, anxious, and tired, and less hostile to other people.

If it is a while since you have done anything active it is best to start gently. If you are not sure whether your heart can take it—that is, if you are aware of having any other of the risk factors—check with your doctor to decide a sensible approach. Otherwise, just try a short, brisk walk—ten minutes to start with—to see how you get on. If you are panting and exhausted at the end of this, you have reached your current threshold. Don't attempt any longer distances until you can cope with this comfortably. If you walk this distance regularly, say on alternate days, you will soon improve. Then you can set yourself a fifteen-minute target, and so on.

The amount to aim for finally, which is thought to maintain us at a good level of fitness, is about four sessions of brisk exercise a week, each of half an hour's duration. This means a pace at which you notice that your heart and breathing rate have speeded up, but which does not make you so out of breath that you can't maintain it for the half-hour. The steady pace and the length of time you keep going are more beneficial than achieving a lightning speed. Choose a type of exercise you enjoy, so that there is a good chance you will want to do it regularly—this is to be a change for life, not just for a limited period. Walking, swimming, cycling, team sports and gym workouts are all worth considering. Ask your friends if they want to participate as well, because a social aspect to the exercise will make it much easier to maintain.

Diabetes

This problem has differing levels of severity and the treatment will vary accordingly. It is caused by a lack of the hormone insulin, which is produced by the pancreas when the level of sugar in the bloodstream is high. It stimulates the uptake of sugar from the bloodstream into the cells of the body where it is used as a fuel to power most of the work that those cells perform. The reduction in the amount of insulin made may be only partial, or it may be complete. For those who still make a little insulin, treatment may consist of a special diet limiting their intake of sugar, so that their blood sugar level never gets too high. Those with a more serious deficiency may need medication in tablet form, and for people who have lost the ability to make any insulin, an injection of it will be necessary, in conjunction with a diet that regulates the amount and timing of their carbohydrate intake.

Most diabetes sufferers check their own sugar levels regularly with either a blood or urine test. It is necessary to keep blood sugar levels within the healthy range to feel well, and also to reduce the risk of cardiovascular disease: people with high blood sugar levels have higher rates of heart attacks.

The main symptoms of diabetes are unexplained tiredness, passing excessive amounts of urine, possibly accompanied by extreme thirst (to make up the loss of water from the body). A simple urine test will indicate whether diabetes is the cause. If you are diagnosed as diabetic it is most important to keep to the treatment your doctor prescribes.

Stress

This is a word we frequently hear applied to modern life. Does that mean that our ancestors never had problems to contend with? On the contrary, life was short and hard for most previous generations, but nowadays we have different problems to cope with, and different situations in which to react. Our bodies come complete with a system of responses which served us well for getting out of trouble in the distant past. This is called the 'fight or flight' response, and is activated by a particular part of the nervous system. It is not under voluntary or conscious control, and so is within what is termed the 'autonomic' nervous system—it functions without our being aware of it. But we are only too aware of its consequences. Fight or flight was the way our ancestors reacted to threats—you either held your ground and tried to overcome the danger, or ran away as fast as you could. Both options required the maximum strength you were capable of, and the changes triggered in your body made you capable of just that. Think of how you feel when you are nervous: the changes include rapid breathing and heart rate, muscle tension (in preparation for action), and rapid mental activity. What is going on below the level of your awareness is that your blood is circulating faster and at higher pressure and is directed to your muscles, your airways are opened up to get more oxygen into your lungs, and your adrenal glands are producing hormones: adrenalin to reinforce the action of the nervous system and cortisol to release stores of fat into your bloodstream to fuel your exertions.

This system worked well when the threats were of a physical nature, and of limited duration. It still does work for people in dangerous situations, by enhancing their performance at the time. After the danger has been dealt with, the nervous system should calm down and return to normal functioning with no difficulty.

But think how unsuitable those reactions are if the problem is connected with work deadlines, tension with other members of staff, worry about finances, redundancy, your marriage, and so on—the fight or flight response occurs in these circumstances just as it does against physical danger. In these situations, particularly if you don't exercise to use the body in the way it is prepared

51

for, you run the risk of developing health problems, including cardiovascular disease.

This tendency has been found to be associated with one personality trait in particular. The term 'Type A personality' was first used in America to describe the sort of person who was very ambitious and competitive, impatient and intolerant of other people. The frequency of cardiovascular disease in people of different characters has been studied and it has been shown that it is overwhelmingly Type As who have the greatest incidence. But it seems that not all the Type A characteristics carry the same risk. It is particularly the characteristics of hostility and aggressiveness to other people that cause the problems. This is not hard to understand: confrontational behaviour will automatically turn on the fight or flight response, and in someone who behaves like this frequently it will be occurring too often for good health.

It is possible to change this characteristic, for the sake of one's health. Various types of relaxation therapy and psychotherapy aim to help people 'unlearn' it, for the benefit of the individual and doubtless also for the rest of the family. Other stress-reducing factors have also been identified. One is belonging to a particular social group in which you feel at home, such as a caring family or a church. The feeling of being accepted and valued, of having friends you can trust and keeping to a predictable and stable way of life, seem to reduce the harmful impact of other types of stress. Even a pet helps keep you more stress-free: research has shown that pet owners have somewhat lower rates of fat and cholesterol in their blood, and lower blood pressure, than non pet owners.

Smoking

The dangers of this habit must be known to everyone in the Western world. Cigarette companies are even facing court cases nowadays, taken out by people whose health has been destroyed. We know about its effect on the lungs, but the effect on the circulation is less familiar. Of the cocktail of toxic substances within tobacco, it is the nicotine and the carbon monoxide that have the worst effects. Nicotine acts to constrict the blood vessels, resulting in a rise in blood pressure as the diameter of the tubes is narrowed, and the amount of blood getting through may be reduced. If the flow is already reduced by partial blockage of the vessel due to arteriosclerosis, this will worsen the condition. Nicotine also speeds up blood clotting which, in vessels that are already unhealthy, increases the risk of thrombosis.

Carbon monoxide reduces the oxygen-carrying capacity of the blood, by competing with oxygen for the carrier sites on haemoglobin in the red blood cells. The main problem with this is that, whereas oxygen can be both taken up and released freely by the haemoglobin, once carbon monoxide has combined with it there is no reversal. So there is a permanent reduction of the oxygen-carrying potential. In a person who already has circulation problems, this further reduction of oxygen adds to the risk of severe symptoms.

Smoking is also the prime avoidable cause of the formation of harmful substances called *free radicals*. These are coming to the attention of the medical profession and the public as they are implicated in the development of numerous serious diseases. They are basically unstable (and therefore highly reactive) atoms which are by-products of certain processes in the body. They are generally short-lived, as they combine readily but quite randomly with other molecules in the tissues by a reaction called oxidation. Their destructive potential is due to the fact that the oxidised molecule will be permanently altered, and may no longer be able to perform its previous function.

Free radicals are produced by many processes, some of which are essential to normal health, such as the production of energy from the breaking down of glucose within cells. The body has some defence against them in the form of enzymes that can deactivate them and render them harmless. There are also certain vitamins and minerals, known as antioxidants, that can react with them before they do any harm. These include vitamins A, C and E. If too many free radicals are produced, however, they can speed up the ageing rate of the body, increase the risk of cancer, and cause deterioration to the circulation.

So how to stop smoking? There are plenty of techniques to try. If one doesn't work for you, don't let discouragement stop you trying again: any reduction is worth the effort, and stopping completely could mean the difference between living out years of enjoyment or miserable disablement at the end of your life.

Diets for cardiovascular health
This subject has been taken increasingly seriously in the last twenty years. The basic principle is to get back to eating more of the foods for which we are best adapted, and to cut down on those that are highly processed.

The current advice from nutritionists is to eat at least two pieces of fruit a day, along with three portions of fresh vegetables. It is recommended that at least one of the vegetable portions is a green leafy type, either cooked, such as cabbage or broccoli, or raw salad greens. All the root vegetables are excellent, and very underrated. Salads should be eaten in winter as well as summer—as a side dish if not the main course. Apart from lettuce, tomato and cucumber, try finely-grated raw carrot, red, green or yellow peppers, watercress, olives, avocados, vegetable fennel, endive and exotic lettuces, beetroot (but not the pickled type—the plain boiled type is better tasting), and use olive oil in the dressing. There is plenty of evidence that the substances that give the different colours to vegetables all have protective benefits for us—the yellow, orange, red, purple and green pigments all contribute to our health in different ways. So make your meals as colourful as possible and you will be enhancing their health potential.

The other great benefit of fruit and vegetables is the fibre they contain. This does not have a nutritional function: its value is that it remains unabsorbed by the body and therefore stays in the digestive tract, providing the bulk that stimulates the movement of food through the gut. The combination of plenty of fibre in the diet and healthy amounts of exercise should keep everything moving smoothly and briskly, avoiding problems of constipation. If you find that some very high-fibre vegetables upset your digestion, of course avoid them—there will still be plenty that you can eat.

What we should be eating less of are the dairy and flesh foods. These are far more concentrated in nutrients, so we need proportionally less of them than of the much more watery and fibrous vegetable foods. A relatively small amount will give us all we need in the way of nutrition; in larger amounts they become a liability rather than an asset. The two major nutrients in animal products are protein and fats. Protein is a vital constituent of our diet, as it provides the building blocks for growth in children and repair of damage in adults. Adults need about 60 grammes (two and a half ounces) of protein a day to fulfil this need. If we eat more than we need, it is stored as body fat.

The fat in red meat and dairy foods is mainly in the form of the highly undesirable saturated fat. Fatty cuts of beef for stewing or mince are high in saturated fats, as are lamb chops, roast lamb, braised spare ribs of pork and fatty gammon. It is this type of fat that is associated with increased cholesterol levels and therefore cardio-vascular disease. And, of course, it is very rich in calories, so if you don't exercise to use up what you consume, your weight will steadily increase. It is easy to reduce your intake of saturated fats by changing to semi-skimmed or skimmed milk, low fat cheeses (including Mozzarella, feta, cottage cheese and reduced-fat hard cheeses such as Cheddar or Edam), and the leanest cuts of red meat, or by eating poultry (not roasted) and fish (not fried) instead.

High blood pressure
This condition, also called hypertension, requires medical diagnosis and assessment. If your reading is above 140/90 your doctor may decide to prescribe medication to reduce the risk of strokes and heart attacks. The cause of the problem varies: in some people it can be an inherited tendency; it may be connected with stress, it can be a consequence of kidney disease or glandular problems, or aggravated by obesity. In some cases a specific cause may not be apparent. It is often associated with arteriosclerosis, though which is the cause and which the effect is not known. Either condition can be present without the other.

Hypertension can be seen as a disease in itself, as many sufferers have symptoms including headaches, dizziness and palpitations. If you suffer from these, visit your doctor for a check on your blood pressure. Hypertension can be present without causing symptoms, but even so it is still a risk factor and medical treatment is necessary. You can enhance the benefits of treatment by reducing excess body weight, through changing your diet and by taking more exercise (with medical advice about what is suitable).

Cholesterol

Most people have heard of cholesterol and know that too much of it can cause circulatory problems. But it is only when difficulties occur with the mechanisms for its regulation, or when the system is overloaded by dietary cholesterol, that these problems develop. One could get the impression from all the adverse news about cholesterol that it is a harmful substance. In fact, it is vitally important for good health—in the right amount. For most people in previous generations it usually was in the right amount.

It is needed as part of the outer membrane of every cell in our bodies. It is also the starter substance for a range of important hormones, including oestrogen and progestogen in women, and testosterone in men. There are three factors that contribute to the amount of cholesterol in the blood: what we take in with our daily food, what is manufactured internally by our liver, and what is excreted by the body (a task also performed by the liver). There has always been individual variation, and a few people have inborn problems with control of cholesterol, due to diseases affecting the amount made or excreted by the liver. The great problem for us nowadays, however, is the huge increase in the amount of cholesterol and fats we take in with our food. This upsets the overall control mechanisms, resulting in higher than desirable cholesterol levels for the majority of the adult population.

Like fats, cholesterol does not mix with water. Because of this, when it is transported in the blood it is combined with certain proteins to form *lipoprotein* (meaning fat plus protein), which enables fats and cholesterol to be dispersed throughout the bloodstream. There are different types of lipoprotein that contain differing proportions of fat to protein, and the relative amounts of these in the blood are very significant for our health.

To understand the problems, we need to know how cholesterol is carried around the body by the various types of lipoprotein transport systems. There are three main types of these lipoproteins: very low density lipoproteins (VLDLs) which have a high amount of fat in them and relatively little protein, low density lipoproteins (LDLs) with a slightly lower ratio of fat to protein, and high density lipoproteins (HDLs) with significantly less fat to protein. The lower the amount of fat, the higher the amount of protein and density of the lipoprotein. After a meal has been digested, the fats from it are combined into VLDLs by the liver and released into the bloodstream to be transported to the fat-burning and fat-storing tissues. Obviously, the more fat that has been eaten, the more VLDLs there will be in the blood. These contain a small amount of cholesterol as well. After the fat-using tissues have taken in the fats from the VLDLs these become LDLs, and now have a higher ratio of cholesterol in them. This is the form of lipoprotein that causes most problems by depositing the cholesterol in the walls of the blood vessels. So the more fat we eat, the more VLDLs we make, and the more dangerous LDLs we are left with. For most people, the LDLs form about 60–70 per cent of their total cholesterol count. HDLs form about 20–30 per cent, and the VLDLs make up the remainder. These percentages are not permanently fixed: change in diet has brought them about, and reversing those changes can correct them again.

The third type of lipoprotein, thought to be beneficial in that it can protect against the development of cardiovascular disease, is the HDLs. They can take cholesterol from the LDLs and transport it back to the liver from where it is excreted into the digestive tract in the bile. The more HDLs we have, the easier the liver's job of getting rid of excess cholesterol.

How important is the contribution of raised cholesterol levels to the risk of cardiovascular disease? The first theories about this were put forward in the 1930s, and evidence has been accumulating steadily over the last thirty years. Long-term studies have been conducted on large numbers of people and have shown conclusively that, even if other risk factors are at a low level, blood cholesterol levels give an accurate prediction of the risk of developing cardiovascular disease later in life (though how much later cannot be predicted). The current thinking is that for every one per cent drop in a person's blood cholesterol level there is a two per cent drop in the risk of coronary heart disease. As changes in diet and other factors can achieve a cholesterol reduction of 25 per cent, this means that a person's risk of cardiovascular disease can be cut by 50 per cent—a dramatically more hopeful outlook for one's later years of life. It is thought that the process of arteriosclerosis can definitely be slowed down, and possibly halted completely or even reversed by such cholesterol reduction.

If you have a blood cholesterol test you will be given the result expressed as a figure which will fall between the extremes of 3 and 9. Low readings, between 4.00 and 5.2, are considered to be healthy and desirable. Moderately high levels are between 5.2 and 6.5, and above this is the undesirably high range. Readings above 7 are thought to require some type of treatment to bring them down. In the UK 60 per cent of the population have readings above 5.2 – the average is 5.9. Therefore most people would benefit by taking steps to reduce their levels.

You may be thinking that a total cholesterol test could be misleading in that it covers both harmful LDLs and beneficial HDLs without giving the proportion of either, and you will be right. The interpretation of total cholesterol, and the risk it presents, has to be made in the light of an individual's way of life. In someone who is slim, takes plenty of aerobic exercise and eats a suitable diet the proportion of HDL is likely to be much higher than in someone who is overweight, inactive and fond of high-fat foods. To clarify this situation, a more discriminating test is available to check the relative levels of LDLs and HDLs.

If you haven't already been tested for cholesterol you may be wondering whether you should ask your doctor about this. Give some thought to the other risk factors, and if any of them are obviously positive a cholesterol reading will help to clarify your degree of risk of cardiovascular disease. If your cholesterol level is above the desirable range you should make changes that will lower it. Look at this as a beneficial change for everyone in your family: remember that the lower the cholesterol, the better their chance of enjoying cardiovascular health in the future. As the development of fatty streaks in blood vessels is known to start in childhood, getting used to a healthy diet at an early age will pay off later (though low-fat milk should not be introduced until the age of five—full-fat milk is too valuable nutritionally to be replaced before this).

The following dietary changes will help to reduce only the harmful LDLs, so that the ratio of HDL/LDL will improve. Incidentally, the changes should also help to protect against cancers of the colon and breast, which seem to be connected with fat and fibre balance in the diet.

Your main objective should be to reduce the amounts of saturated fats (found in red meat, whole milk, cheese, butter, hardened margarines, coconut oil and palm oil as used in processed foods, and cocoa butter in chocolate) and to increase unsaturated fats (found in oily fish such as salmon, herring and mackerel, and in vegetable oils, especially olive and peanut oils). The influences these fats have on cholesterol levels is greater than the effect of consuming cholesterol itself. Saturated fats raise cholesterol twice as much as unsaturated fats lower it, so you need to cut down on these rather than just increasing the amount of unsaturated fat you eat. If you have an undesirably high cholesterol level you will see a quicker improvement if you cut down on cholesterol intake as well. You will be doing this automatically by cutting down on sources of saturated fat, as these are also the high-cholesterol foods, but in addition reduce your intake of eggs to a maximum of two or three a week, and reduce organ meats like liver and kidneys. Judging by the results of tests where only cholesterol itself was reduced, it seems that there is a wide variation in the way people respond: in some it causes a significant reduction in blood cholesterol levels, whilst in others there is virtually no resulting difference. It is thought that a reduction can be valuable to most people, however, because there may be a connection between dietary intake and an increased clotting tendency in the blood, independent of actual cholesterol levels.

The other important change is to increase the amount of fruit and vegetables you eat. This will raise your intake of vitamins and minerals, and especially of fibre. Extra fibre can also be found in whole grain cereals and pulses.

The amount of coffee you drink could be having an effect on your cholesterol levels—there is some (but conflicting) evidence that decaffeinated is the worst type, with percolated and cafetière next, and filtered real coffee the least harmful. Advice on alcohol consumption is similarly controversial. Whilst there is evidence that a small intake of up to two units a day (the equivalent of two glasses of wine, two measures of spirits or one pint of beer) may help lower cholesterol, larger amounts are undesirable as other risks outweigh the possible advantages. If you are a non-drinker, don't start just to help your cholesterol levels—work harder at the other changes instead.

Two other important aspects of cholesterol-lowering are exercise and weight-loss for those who are overweight. This shows how closely related matters of nutrition, circulation and exercise are, and that when one factor in our way of life moves away from health, others are affected too. Aerobic exercise has been found to raise HDLs. Thus, in combination with suitable dietary changes, regular exercise can bring about a beneficial change in the ratio of HDL to LDL. And in overweight people who have come down in weight through a combination of suitable diet and exercise, LDL levels themselves have been found to be reduced.

The improvement in cholesterol levels that is achieved by making these changes will vary from one person to another: we are all individuals, and have individual responses. Whilst one person may achieve a comparatively rapid and successful result, another may be discouraged by finding only a small change for all his or her efforts. If this happens, there is another approach that can help the situation before one needs to resort to orthodox medication. A supplement of garlic alongside the other changes could help enormously.

CHAPTER 6

Ginkgo and Garlic—the Specifics

As we have seen, diseases of the circulation, and asthma, owe much to our modern lifestyle, and going back to more natural and traditional habits of eating and exercise can help restore health. But there are other natural strategies that can also help: our herbs, ginkgo and garlic. The first part of this chapter suggests what problems they can help with, and the second part, written for the curious, explains why. It is of necessity far more technical than any previous chapter, but has been written as simply as possible in the belief that many readers will find it of interest.

We know that the way cardiovascular disease develops is a slow, unnoticeable downhill path. The process starts in youth, and the results don't show themselves until the problems are so far advanced that a return to full health is at best very difficult. Until recently, by the time you realised you were unhealthy it was too late to do much about it, except to try to limit future problems. Now, however, the situation is less bleak. The effort put into researching the causes of the epidemic has paid off, resulting in the understanding about risk factor assessment discussed in the previous chapter. An assessment of each of the risk factors in your particular case can help you work out your individual risk likelihood, and by taking steps to adjust your way of life you can improve your chances of staying healthy in the future. You are able to avoid the blight of cardiovascular disease because you have the knowledge about it that the previous generation lacked. And as well as your own efforts at change, garlic and ginkgo can work

61

for your benefit. By combining the changes in your lifestyle with the use of natural remedies you will enhance the success of each.

Of course, taking ginkgo and garlic for a problem (especially if there are as yet no signs of it) is rather different from trying to change your way of living. How do you know when you really need them? There is no specific answer to this, except by making a realistic assessment of your risks: the more factors for which you are positive, the greater the chance that you will benefit from taking either garlic or ginkgo, or both.

They are relevant to any stage of the problem. Before obvious disease has developed, they can both be safely taken as a preventative treatment. You might think there is no point in taking them if there is no sign of trouble, but we know now that in the developed world, the changes in lifestyle associated with cardiovascular disease start to cause harmful changes quite early in life. Post mortem studies have shown deterioration in the blood vessels even in teenagers, and the more a child eats in the way of saturated fats, and the less exercise he or she takes, the earlier the age at which the problems develop. Of course the first step to better health is to change your exercise and eating habits, but there is no reason why you should not introduce garlic into your diet as part of your dietary changes. It could prevent the problems from getting a lot worse. In fact, as fashions in food are changing, many more youngsters nowadays are enjoying the pungent tastes of Mediterranean and Asian foods, and so will grow up accepting a wide range of exotic additions to their diet.

Many people have blood pressure and cholesterol levels that are not obviously high, but may be marginally so. Such people don't want to be 'medicalised' into facing the rest of their lives on drug treatments if they can help it: they want to keep control of their own health. A combination of diet, exercise and supplementation with natural remedies (in European countries, both ginkgo and garlic are classed as dietary treatments) can really pay off here, helping to prevent the person from crossing the border into a diagnosed condition of illness. Where there is evidence of disease, ginkgo and garlic can help to improve the situation, and enable a return to health in some measure. Even where there is advanced disease, although other treatments may also be necessary, ginkgo and garlic will still both help to avoid the risk of the serious consequences of cardiovascular or respiratory disease occurring. **If you are already taking medication from your doctor, tell him or her that you are considering trying ginkgo and garlic. It is important that all aspects of your treatment are known to your doctor.**

To illustrate the uses of ginkgo and garlic, let's take the hypothetical case of a man (or it could equally well be a woman) who at age sixty has started to have mild symptoms of cardiovascular problems. A review of the risk factors will indicate how these might have developed. Our patient has, say, one parent who had a heart attack—so there could be an inherited tendency to heart disease. He has got out of the habit of taking much exercise, since he drives a car and has plenty of labour-saving gadgets around the house. Most people slow down and reduce the amount of activity they do as they get older, seeing this as taking a well-earned rest towards the end of a busy life. As a result, our friend's weight has been creeping up in recent years, and he is becoming apple-shaped around the middle. Retirement from a stressful managerial job is coming up soon, offering him the opportunity to spend more time enjoying all the things that he hasn't had time for previously. His meals have consisted of the typical British food: occasional fried breakfasts, meat or cheese sandwiches at lunchtime, and meat and vegetables in the evening. He used to smoke, but gave up recently after a severe chest infection. He has been troubled by being increasingly out of breath when walking uphill, and finds at the same time that he now has to stop and rest to relieve the cramp developing in his calf muscles. This makes him less inclined to do much exercise: he feels he must be getting too old and the cramps are an unpleasant reminder of this.

He visits his doctor, who finds that his blood pressure and cholesterol levels are moderately high. Thus there is some evidence that he is at risk of more severe problems developing in the future if he doesn't do something to change his habits now: most of the risk factors are present to some degree. He may find that his mental faculties are becoming less sharp, with memory loss, and difficulties with concentration and problem-solving. If he developed severe problems with circulation to his brain, his family could find his personality changed and his ability to look after himself greatly diminished. He takes the problem seriously, remembering the effect that his father's heart problems had on the family.

He is greatly cheered by the doctor's assurance that there are several changes he himself can make, which in themselves will almost certainly help. At this stage these can be put into practice and his improvement assessed after a few months: if they are successful, he may not need to have any medication for the condition. The doctor's advice is to go on a cholesterol-lowering diet and to start a programme of exercise, geared to his present state of fitness. The suggestions given by the doctor are very similar to those in chapter 5, but tailored specifically to his needs. If he can keep to them and practise them regularly, the benefits should be both an enhanced feeling of health and fitness, and a reduction in blood pressure and cholesterol levels. Most people will gain these benefits, but a few may not: everyone is different and the degree of improvement will vary from one person to another. What else can be done to help?

Ginkgo and garlic both have a role to play. Garlic can help to lower blood cholesterol, and will work alongside the cholesterol-lowering diet. It helps to reduce the amount of harmful low-density lipoproteins in the blood, which are closely connected with high cholesterol. It also works with the exercise programme in this respect, as exercise helps to shift the other side of the balance, by increasing the amount of beneficial high-density lipoprotein. This means that garlic is useful in just about every problem of the circulation where the build-up of atheroma or arteriosclerosis is involved, such as our friend's leg cramps when he walks too far. It can also help, along with exercise, to reduce the high blood pressure, particularly in people who have associated problems of high blood cholesterol and fat levels, and it will help to protect against the harmful consequences of these conditions whilst they are improving, by lowering the risk of thromboses or embolism. The same effect can be enhanced by ginkgo. This is another potent remedy to keep the blood thin, in a different way from garlic, but having the same overall result. The risk of thrombosis and embolism, and therefore of heart attacks and strokes, is significantly reduced. Other risks, such as damage to the brain from impaired blood supply, will also be reduced—garlic helps prevent the initial problem and ginkgo protects against the consequences of it.

Less severe problems with the circulation can also respond to ginkgo and garlic. Garlic, as mentioned previously, has traditionally been considered a 'warming' remedy. Ginkgo is known to improve the flow of blood through the smallest blood vessels, the capillaries. Many people suffer from cold hands and feet or chilblains in the winter. This is not necessarily a sign of any disease of the circulation: it is more likely to be a characteristic of the individual's general constitution. It is an unpleasant experience, though, and ginkgo and garlic may well help to prevent it. More severe symptoms may be diagnosed as Raynaud's syndrome, and both ginkgo and garlic can help by improving the blood flow to the hands and feet.

People suffering from insufficiency of blood to the brain are very likely to benefit from taking both remedies. This problem is given a much higher priority for treatment in Europe than in the UK. It is very difficult to diagnose the main cause of the loss of mental powers in elderly people, but there is likely to be at least some degree of insufficient blood supply. Ginkgo and garlic can help here to improve the circulation to the brain, thus reducing symptoms such as loss of memory and ability to concentrate, dizziness, headaches and depression. But they will have less effect if the main cause is something other than insufficient blood supply.

Tinnitus is a distressing condition that can be one aspect of the more general problem of insufficiency of blood supply to the brain in elderly people, or it can affect those of a much younger age as an isolated symptom that occurs suddenly, sometimes accompanied by dizziness and deafness. The combination of actions shown by ginkgo and garlic is likely to help restore the supply of blood and prevent the damage to nerve cells that may occur when tinnitus develops. Another disease of which tinnitus is just one symptom is Ménière's syndrome. This is characterised by severe dizziness and difficulty in balancing, vomiting, and noises in the ears or head. Although no clinical trials have been held so far, there are case histories indicating the value of ginkgo (and theoretically garlic as well) in the treatment of Ménière's disease.

For an asthma sufferer, the value of taking garlic is that it reduces the respiratory infections to which he or she may be prone. An infection causes extra irritation in the airways, provoking the production of even more mucus than usual, thus adding to the obstruction to breathing. It is also likely to trigger more constriction in the muscles lining the airways. Garlic is a natural anti-infective remedy which at the right dose will reduce the risk of infections.

Ginkgo is more likely to help by reducing the severity of the asthma symptoms themselves. So far, no single treatment can completely control asthma, although various medications given as inhalers can alleviate the worst of the symptoms. However, there are good reasons for believing that ginkgo may help. Because it is thought that there are multiple factors involved in the causes of asthma, it would be misleading to suggest that ginkgo by itself can cure the problem. Having said that, it is thought that ginkgo can make some contribution to the control of certain types of asthma. Although no clinical trials have yet been carried out, undoubtedly some will take place in the near future to clarify whether or not this is the case. In the meantime, there is no reason why anyone suffering from asthma should not try ginkgo to see if there is a benefit to be gained from it. There will be no conflict with asthma medication that has been prescribed by a doctor (but do tell her or him), and this should be continued as prescribed.

Hay fever is caused by a chain of reactions similar to those that cause asthma. The main areas affected are in the eyes, nose and throat rather than in the lungs, and because there is less muscle tissue here the response is mainly inflammation (the main symptoms are itching and profuse watery catarrh produced by the membranes) in the mucous membranes covering the surfaces that are exposed to the allergens. Hay fever is the classic summer problem caused by a reaction to plant pollens, but the same reaction can be caused by fungus spores in the autumn, or by animal fur or feathers at any time of the year. All types are further candidates for the ginkgo and garlic treatment. As with asthma, there have been no clinical trials to check the theory yet, but there is no reason why hay fever sufferers should not try the two remedies to make their own assessment of their effectiveness. It will be interesting to see how their efficacy compares with the antihistamines that are the usual treatment for these problems.

Research is showing that some other health problems may benefit from ginkgo and garlic. Psoriasis is a common distressing and so far incurable skin disease characterised by inflammation and increased speed of production and shedding of the cells in the top layer of the skin. In theory the inflammation which produces the irritation and red appearance of the skin could be eased by both remedies. Clinical trials to check this have not yet been carried out, but sufferers may like to try it for themselves.

Pre-menstrual syndrome is apparently unrelated to the diseases already mentioned, but it is another problem where at least some of the symptoms have been shown to respond to ginkgo. Women who have particular problems with fluid retention and tenderness in the breasts before their menstrual period may find that these are improved by ginkgo. Other symptoms connected with fluid retention elsewhere, such as abdominal bloating and loss of concentration (possibly associated with slight fluid retention in the brain), could also be reduced.

HOW THE REMEDIES WORK

Having discovered what ginkgo and garlic can be used for, you may wonder how they work. This has been researched extensively in the last ten years. Numerous papers on the constituents and actions have been published, but it cannot be claimed that everything about the remedies is scientifically understood as yet.

However, this does not invalidate the results of the clinical trials in which ginkgo and garlic have been separately tested (see chapter 10), or prevent European doctors valuing ginkgo so highly that it is one of their most frequently prescribed remedies for circulation problems. Both remedies are great examples of the principle that herbs cannot be reduced to one 'active constituent'. I hope that, because of their undoubted value in the treatment of cardiovascular problems, they will help to bridge the long-held differences between orthodox and herbal approaches.

Research into ginkgo has revealed at least 140 distinct chemical substances in different parts of the plant, many of which are beneficial medicinally. The main therapeutic constituents of ginkgo leaves are in two distinct classes: *phenols* and *terpenoids*.

Phenols are a huge group of substances, so named because of their similarity in structure to the disinfectant phenol. They occur widely in plants, fungi and bacteria, and have wide-ranging effects on humans. We cannot manufacture them in our bodies, so to get their benefit we must consume them from plant sources. Beneficial phenols include salicylic acid (closely-related to aspirin), and vanillin, which gives the characteristic taste to vanilla pods, and the tannins that give witch hazel its soothing, cooling action. Similar substances in grapes and red wine have been found to have anti-viral properties.

So what are phenols? They all have a common structure, a ring of six carbon atoms at their centre. To get the ring shape, the six carbons each bond to two other carbons in the ring, and to one other atom (it is this part that confers on the phenol its particular reactions and properties). Each carbon in the ring makes one double bond with one other carbon, resulting in a very strong and stable ring structure.

Where a substance consists of more than one six-carbon ring, it is called a polyphenol. The important polyphenols in ginkgo are those of a sub-group called *flavonoids*. These are the largest group of plant phenols, and there are many examples of them, such as the red and yellow pigments that colour many fruits and vegetables. We consume numerous different flavonoids every day from the plants in our diet. The name 'flavonoid' comes from the Latin word *flavus*, meaning yellow. A closely-related group, the anthocyanidins, gives many flowers, fruit and vegetables their red, purple and blue colours (which are also known to benefit our health in other ways). The ginkgo flavonoids are chemically bonded to sugars, resulting in a combination called 'flavonoid glycosides'. On average, ginkgo leaves contain from 0.5 per cent to 1 per cent of flavonoid glycosides.

Terpenoid substances in ginkgo are based on a five-carbon structure called an isoprene unit. These can combine to form various shapes, including rings and chains. Double units, called monoterpenes, give rise to numerous substances found in plant oils (which give the characteristic fragrances to aromatic plants such as mints, pines, thyme, rosemary and so on). Three isoprene units form a sesquiterpene (meaning 'one-and-a-half terpenes'), and one of these, known as *bilobalide*, is one of the active substances in ginkgo. When another isoprene unit is added to sesquiterpenes, a diterpene is formed. A number of these, known as *ginkgolides* A, B, C, J and M, are also active substances in ginkgo leaves. The amount in leaf samples varies greatly, at most being about 0.1 per cent.

Although it contains some monoterpenes, ginkgo could not be described as strong-smelling. In comparison, anyone who has used garlic knows that it is downright pungent. The active constituents, even though they have a similar action to those of ginkgo, are completely different in structure. The discovery of the active constituents (described in chapter 1) identified them as the pungent-smelling, sulphur-containing substances, including *allicin*, *diallyl disulphide* and *ajoene*. The smell is common to many sulphur-containing plant substances. Some, such as mustard, also have an acrid taste. This is caused by the slightly irritating effect of the constituents on the mucous membranes lining the mouth and nasal cavities.

Other constituents of garlic include various terpenes in the oil, and the non-oily fraction contains vitamins, minerals and fats, as would be expected in the part of the plant that acts as a food store over the winter, to nourish the new growth that will be produced the following year.

Our ancestors had no way of analysing plants to arrive at this knowledge, and it is remarkable that even so they discerned the benefits of ginkgo and garlic, and used them therapeutically. One can only suppose that, because of the critical need in the past to find the most successful plant medicines available, a lot of very close attention was devoted to observing the influence of different plants on people's health. Nowadays we have the advantage of being able to account scientifically for most of that beneficial effect.

In ginkgo, the benefit lies with various effects that the flavonoids and terpenes have on mechanisms involved with blood-clotting and inflammation. As described in chapter 2, the 'stickiness' of blood is due to the activity of the platelets it contains. These are activated by contact with areas of damage on the walls of the blood vessels, either when there is a breach of the vessel wall (which is the healthy function of preventing blood-loss into the tissues, and repairing the breach) or when there is atheroma or arteriosclerosis (when the reaction is harmful in that it adds to the existing problem). One of the chemicals produced by both the cells that line the blood vessels and by circulating white cells and platelets themselves, which triggers this reaction in the platelets, is called *Platelet Activating Factor* (PAF). This is released when there is an abnormality of the vessel wall, either due to a rupture of the vessel or to atheroma or arteriosclerosis. When PAF is released, it causes the platelets to become stickier. They change shape from discs to spheres and with other platelets form a clump that connects with the damaged part of the blood vessel. They release numerous substances, including a fatty acid (a component of fats) known as *arachidonic acid*. This is quickly broken down to other substances, by various enzymes, and the products are closely involved with the development of blood-clotting, allergic reactions and other inflammatory reactions.

One of the products of arachidonic acid breakdown is called *thromboxane A2*. This itself stimulates further platelet activation, causing a great increase in the scale of the reactions. It also causes constriction of the blood vessel, by increasing the contraction of muscle fibres in the vessel wall. This is a very helpful reaction if the cause of the problem is a break in the vessel wall: it cuts down on the amount of blood lost before clotting takes place. But if the reaction is due to atheroma, it is another disadvantage because it means that even less blood is going to flow along the vessel to the local tissues. So the more thromboxane formed, the greater the number of platelets that become involved in the process, and the larger the resulting platelet plug.

In healthy blood vessels, the formation of platelet plugs is decreased by another substance produced by the cells lining the blood vessels. *Prostacyclin*, also made from arachidonic acid and released into the bloodstream, helps to reduce platelet activation and prevents constriction of the muscles in the vessel walls. The overall balance between the amounts of thromboxane and prostacyclin determines whether or not platelet clumping and clot formation will proceed. If the walls of the blood vessels are smooth and undamaged, prostacyclin dominates and prevents platelet activation.

When arachidonic acid is produced by platelets, it leads to the formation of another group of substances called *leukotrienes*. These cause inflammation and allergic reactions, including asthma. They induce contraction in the muscles in the walls of the airways. One cause of the formation of leukotrienes is the release of PAF in the membranes lining the airways: the cells here, like those lining the blood vessels, will produce it under certain conditions. When PAF is released it triggers certain cells of the immune system into activity, resulting in inflammation. More immune cells are attracted to the lining of the airway, where they produce a range of substances, including PAF itself, so that the scale of the problem increases. As well as the direct immune cell reactions, platelet activation and arachidonic acid are involved, resulting in the formation of leucotrienes. These cause swelling and damage in the lining of the airways, leading to the production of thick, jelly-like mucus, and muscular constriction resulting in narrowing of the airways and obstruction to normal breathing.

The development of inflammation also results in the production of harmful free radicals. These were described in chapter 5 as a risk to health, being implicated in circulatory disease, mental impairment and cancer. The production of PAF and free radicals is thought to lead to the reperfusion damage to brain cells that occurs after temporary occurrences of cerebral insufficiency (see p. 40 for a fuller explanation).

Any substances that block PAF activity, and prevent the chain reactions it causes, will thus be most beneficial to people suffering from arteriosclerosis, 'sticky' blood, asthma, cerebrovascular problems and the other diseases we have already discussed. This is just what the ginkgo flavonoids and terpenes are able to do. There could be several stages along the chain of events from platelet activation or arachidonic acid production to the final disease state where the flavonoids might exert their influence. They might block the pathways by which both thromboxane and the leucotrienes are formed. They seem to stimulate the production of prostacyclin, and so reduce the risk of platelet activation. Ginkgo also functions as an antioxidant, and so protects the body from a wide range of possible damage from free radicals. The terpenes have a very specific action: they block the sites where PAF latches on to the cells that are involved in the reactions. There is a precise fit between the shape of a molecule such as PAF and the complementary shape of the site on a cell membrane into which it slots, rather like a lock and key. A molecule that doesn't fit exactly will not trigger the same reaction in the cell. The ginkgolides have a shape similar enough to PAF to be able to latch onto the membrane, but as they are not identical they don't trigger the same reactions. The result is that by occupying the receptor sites on the cell membrane, they prevent PAF doing so, and thus prevent the cell's reactions from being triggered.

Garlic too helps to reduce platelet activity, blood stickiness, blood vessel constriction and blood pressure. It also helps to reduce the level of fats circulating in the blood, and this has the effect of reducing cholesterol levels. The sulphur-containing constituents are thought to be the active principles, with the cholesterol-lowering action specifically possessed by diallyl disulphide. It is thought to work by altering the balance between the formation of fats (which is reduced) and the breakdown of existing fats (which is increased). The outcome of this is that there are fewer of the harmful low density lipoproteins which take fats to storage cells, and more of the beneficial type that transports cholesterol from the tissues to the liver to be excreted. The cholesterol level therefore drops. Allicin and ajoene are both thought to be involved in the reduction of platelet activation. They could prevent the production of thromboxane by inhibiting the enzymes involved, or affect the membranes of the platelets to prevent the release of arachidonic acid; or they could prevent the uptake of calcium into the platelets that is necessary for activation processes. Allicin is probably the main active constituent here, though the other sulphur-containing substances may have some activity: ajoene has also been shown to block PAF receptors and thus inhibit platelet activation, preventing them from clumping and releasing arachidonic acid. It is thought to work by its action on the outer membrane surrounding the platelet. It may also increase the effect of prostacyclin in preventing platelet activation.

The other great benefit of garlic, for asthma sufferers, is its ability to help prevent chest infections. It is known to destroy infections caused by numerous bacteria including staphylococcus, and fungi such as aspergillus. In laboratory conditions it has also been shown to work against some types of herpes virus (the type responsible for causing cold sores) and some types of influenza virus. Here again, allicin is thought to be the main active constituent.

We can now compare the actions of ginkgo and garlic with the best-known orthodox remedy that is recommended to keep the blood thin—aspirin. The full name of the chemical is acetylsalicylic acid. Both the chemical and common names are associated with its 'herbal' origin: for hundreds of years herbalists were using preparations made from meadowsweet (whose former botanical name was *Spiraea*, from which the name aspirin was derived, though it is now reclassified as *Filipendula*) and willow bark (botanical name: *Salix*, from which salicylic was derived) for treating the pain and inflammation of conditions like arthritis and rheumatism. Both plants contain phenols very similar to aspirin, as well as many other beneficial constituents. Aspirin itself works in a way similar to ginkgo and garlic. When arachidonic acid is produced by the activated platelets, aspirin will inhibit the action of enzymes that break it down further. Thus it prevents the formation of thromboxane (but also the production of the beneficial prostacyclin in the walls of the blood vessels). It also stops the production of substances called prostaglandins in a wide range of tissues. This may be very helpful in averting the harmful consequences of cardiovascular disease, and also prevents the sensation of pain that prostaglandins trigger. The problem with aspirin is that it has an irritating effect on the stomach. Most people can tolerate this without too much difficulty, but some have a severe reaction that makes it impossible for them to take any aspirin at all. Ginkgo and garlic would be a preferable and equally effective alternative.

When considering its cholesterol-lowering effect, we can compare garlic with numerous orthodox treatments. There are various ways that the orthodox medicines work. One group of them, including cholestyramine, increases the amount of cholesterol that the liver binds to acids which are then excreted into the bile. This is secreted into the digestive tract to contribute to the digestion of fats, and eventually passes out of the body as the brown pigment that gives the characteristic colour to the stools. One problem connected with this is that although it reduces the amount of cholesterol in the blood, it leaves behind the fats that were bound to the cholesterol. There is therefore a risk that it might increase the levels of fat in the blood, which in itself is very undesirable. Some other remedies, known as the clofibrate group, function more to reduce the overall amount of fats in the blood, which results in a lowering of cholesterol as well. A third group, based on nicotinic acid, has the benefit of lowering both cholesterol and fat levels in the blood.

You may wonder why, if these drugs work, there is any need

to consider ginkgo and garlic as alternatives. The answer is that all these treatments have been found to have side-effects. Not everyone will experience these: some people will tolerate the treatments more easily than others. Among the problems that have been recorded are, for the cholestyramine, digestive disturbances and the risk of shortage of the fat-soluble vitamins (vitamins A, D, E and K) and folic acid, which therefore require supplementation. The clofibrate group can cause gallstones, digestive disorders and impotence (due to the body's need for a certain amount of cholesterol to manufacture the sex hormones, including the male hormone testosterone). The nicotinic acid group can cause digestive disorders and an unpleasant flushing and itching of the skin. In the next chapter there is an assessment of the possible side-effects of ginkgo and garlic, which you can compare with the list above.

It is easy to see now that, rather than just the single action of other drugs, both ginkgo and garlic work in multiple ways, as a result of containing multiple active constituents, to help cardiovascular and respiratory problems. We know that ginkgo and garlic together achieve their benefits in five ways: they will help to reduce high blood cholesterol levels, they reduce high blood fat levels in general, they maintain blood fluidity and prevent unhealthy activation of platelets that leads to thrombosis and reduced blood supply, and they reduce the constriction of blood vessels that contributes to high blood pressure. In comparison, the only thing that aspirin does is to prevent platelet activation, thus keeping the blood thin. To get the whole range of benefits that ginkgo and garlic provide, one would have to take several different drug treatments, all with the risk of side-effects.

CHAPTER 7

How to Take the Remedies

Knowing now that the active constituents of ginkgo are found in the leaves, and those of garlic in the bulb, you may wonder what is the best way of taking them to get the most benefit.

If you are lucky enough to have a ginkgo tree growing in your garden you have access to the basic, unprocessed material that goes into the manufacture of ginkgo extracts. You may wonder whether you can use the leaves from this as your own source of consumption. Making teas from the crude herb is certainly the most widespread and traditional way of preparing herbal medicines. The disadvantage is that you will not be able to tell the amounts of active constituents you will be getting from the crude leaves. Research has shown that these vary greatly in individual trees, depending on the age of the tree (the younger ones contain more active constituents than the mature ones) and the time of year. The ginkgolides are present in highest amounts in the autumn, whilst bilobalides are highest in the summer, and decline in the autumn—though the flavonoid content is fairly constant throughout summer and autumn. There is also an even greater unexplained variation between individual trees, which makes it very difficult to suggest the amount to take to get the benefit.

As it has been shown that we need to get a regular intake of the flavonoids and terpenes to benefit from taking ginkgo, and that the amounts of these in the crude herb cannot be guaranteed, there is a fair risk of not getting what you need from the crude, unstandardised herb. This seems to me to be such a disadvantage that I would say that taking a standardised extract is the preferable option. However, there are some points to argue in favour of the crude herb, such as that, although numerous constituents have been identified as being active, there may be yet others, so far unrecognised, that also contribute to the benefits. By taking the whole leaves you will be getting the benefit of everything in them.

As a guide to dosage, if you decide to take them in this form, if the dried leaves contain the highest amount of flavonoids, you need to take 2–3 grammes of them, three times a day. The easiest type of home preparation, which is the universal traditional technique, is to make a infusion with boiling water (very similar to the preparation of Britain's favourite herbal preparation, tea). Place the leaves in a teapot, pour about a third of a pint of boiling water over them and leave them to infuse for five minutes or so. In this time the water will draw out the constituents from the leaves. Strain the liquid off into a cup, flavour it with honey or fruit juice if you want to, and drink.

The more popular way of taking the remedy is in tablet form. There are plenty of different brands available over-the-counter in most health food shops. All the containers should be labelled with information about the contents, but the range of combinations and strengths, and suggested dosages, may be very confusing. There is a wide safe-dose range, and also a wide effective-dose range. As a guideline, for a tablet containing a standardised extract, the suggested daily dose is 120 milligrams. This is the approximate average dosage that has been used in most of the clinical trials. However, evidence shows that the results are dose-dependent— that is, the larger the dose taken, the more pronounced the results. There are cases where people have taken up to 750mg a day and found the results beneficial, and have experienced no adverse effects. In the 120mg recommended dose, the flavonoid component (flavonoids) is 28mg, and the terpene (ginkgolides and bilobalide) component is 7mg. You can choose between taking a 40mg tablet three times a day, or a slow-release 120mg tablet once a day. If the remedy is in the form of the dried herb in capsules, it should have an analysis of constituents on the pack. Take the equivalent dosage to get the same amount of flavonoids and ginkolides/bilobalides as in the tablets.

For garlic, the most straightforward way of taking it is to eat it raw. Although there is the same problem we have with any crude herbal substance—that the amount of active constituents in the particular sample used are unknown (and it has been shown that in garlic cloves these can vary by a factor of ten)—it has the advantage that you are getting the benefit of everything that is found in the whole clove, with nothing lost by processing. It has also been shown in some trials that taking raw garlic gives the most consistently beneficial results—trials using garlic preparations, in comparison, give much more variable results. Bear in mind that cooking food is itself a type of processing; you may use plenty of garlic in cooking, but you will not get the same medicinal benefit because the heat of the cooking process breaks down some component of the active ingredients. In Mediterranean and Eastern countries eating raw garlic is not unusual, but people in Northern Europe seem far less inclined to do it. The smell of it on the breath, which is unavoidable after eating raw garlic (because, after it has been absorbed through the wall of the digestive tract into the circulation, as it is carried in the bloodstream through the lungs, it passes out of the body through the membranes lining the lungs) and to a lesser extent on the skin, is not considered to be pleasant. The best way of avoiding this is to eat the garlic just before going to sleep, and the smell will be gone by the following morning. This applies to any of the odorous garlic products, such as tablets or capsules. It may also help to eat some other aromatic herb such as parsley leaves or fennel seed after the garlic, to reduce the smell.

The amount you need to take depends on the purpose you want it for. Various trials have been carried out with specific doses, and based on these the recommendations are as follows: eating half to one clove a day (between two and three grammes in weight) has been found to reduce total blood cholesterol by about nine per cent in people who have raised cholesterol levels. One clove a day is also the amount that can protect you against catching infections. But if you are using it to fight off an established infection you will need to take a whole clove three times a day to make it effective—this larger dose is necessary to have a successful action against viruses and bacteria.

The other reason why few people take it raw is that it can upset the stomach. This can be avoided by dividing the clove into three sections, and taking one section three times a day, after meals. The smaller dose will be much better tolerated, and will result in the garlic constituents staying in your body for a longer time span than if you took the whole daily dose at once. It can also be mixed with other foods that buffer the irritating effect it might have on the stomach. You can try crushing the clove to a paste and mixing it with honey or plain yogurt, which makes it much more palatable. As a salad dressing mixed with olive oil, balsamic vinegar and aromatic herbs, it is delicious.

There are numerous traditional and modern processes that preserve or extract and concentrate the properties of garlic.

It is possible to buy bottles of the fresh pressed, stabilised juice, manufactured in Germany by the Schoenenberger company. The garlic juice treatment is recommended to be taken for a month only, in combination with other juices such as hawthorn, for the treatment of arteriosclerosis. The dose is 10ml, twice a day, before meals.

The *British Pharmacopoeia* gives a process for producing official Juice of Garlic, also known as Succus Allii. This consists of taking 80 grammes of fresh bruised garlic and pressing out the juice. What remains of the pressed garlic then has 20ml water added to it, and is pressed again. This is repeated until the total amount of liquid pressed out equals 80ml. Then 20ml of 90 per cent proof alcohol is added to this as a preservative. The mixture is left to stand for two weeks, then filtered. The recommended dose is half to three quarters of a teaspoon, three times a day, for its anti-infective properties.

Alternatively, a traditional and palatable preparation can be made by placing 100 grammes of peeled crushed cloves in a crock pot, then pouring over them 400ml of a mixture of equal parts cider vinegar and water. One recipe recommends that if you boil a little caraway and fennel seed in the vinegar before adding it, the pungency of the final syrup will be reduced. Shake the mixture every day for three days, then strain out the remains of the garlic and stir in two tablespoons of honey. Keep this syrup in the fridge once you have made it. The recommended dose is half to one and a half teaspoons, three times a day.

Another traditional way of preserving the effectiveness of garlic in liquid form was to make an alcoholic extract known as a tincture. This was given in the *British Pharmacopoeia* as follows: take one litre of a solution of 45 per cent alcohol (this could be a spirit of 45 per cent proof) and pour it over 200g of crushed cloves. Leave it soaking for two weeks, shaking it every day. The remains of the garlic should be strained off after two weeks. The recommended dose of this is half to three quarters of a teaspoon, three times daily, for its anti-infective properties.

As with ginkgo, you will find numerous brands of tablets and capsules available in health shops. Garlic powder is made into tablets, and capsules contain oil that is made either by extracting it from the clove by steam distillation, or by soaking the clove in oil to draw out its properties (a technique called maceration). Some are processed to give odourless preparations. The difference in processing will result in different amounts of active constituents in the final product. The amount of allicin that the product contains is used as a guide to its likely efficacy. There is some disagreement as to the effectiveness of the oil—for steam-distilled oils and macerated oils the information is not straightforward. Some researchers report that neither is as effective as the fresh clove or dried form—the steam-distillates are said to be about 35 per cent as effective, and macerated oils about 12 per cent, in preventing platelet clumping. There is some research that shows that the best results in the improvement of blood fluidity and clot dissolving are obtained by taking the dried powder rather than any other preparation, but other opinions consider that because the distilled garlic oil is a very concentrated preparation compared with fresh garlic, it is just as effective. Yet another view is that most products, so long as they have the characteristic garlic smell, will be effective. The evidence from clinical trials using garlic oils is inconclusive on these matters.

There is less controversy about the tablets made of dried garlic:

the best quality tablets contain all the constituents necessary to form allicin, and therefore its breakdown products. They are just as effective as the raw clove. But the allicin content in commercial powders varies tremendously, depending on the conditions under which they were produced. Very quick drying prevents the process of allicin formation: the product will have little smell or therapeutic benefits. If the drying takes place more slowly the allicin will have more time to form, and the smell of the product will reflect this. When garlic powder is sold for culinary rather than medical purposes it may be cheaper because it is not the high-allicin content product, so it cannot be guaranteed to give such good results. One suggestion for standardisation is to express the effectiveness of a preparation in terms of its allicin-releasing potential. All types of preparation could be compared for their likely efficacy in this way. Some preparations are now given a measurement of equivalence to allicin, which again is a useful comparison, so check on the container to see how much there is per tablet.

When taking a good-quality garlic powder tablet, the following doses are recommended: research has shown that you need a daily dose of 3.5–5.5mg of allicin (the equivalent of about 600–900mg a day of good quality dried garlic powder) for at least three months to get an effective reduction in blood cholesterol and fat levels. For use as a help in the prevention of infections, the same amount can be taken regularly and indefinitely. To treat an active infection, about three times this amount is required.

The remaining point to consider about our two remedies, without which this account would be incomplete, is the question of side-effects and contraindications.

ARE GINKGO AND GARLIC SAFE TO TAKE?

Although they are extremely effective remedies, both ginkgo and garlic are, for most people, free of side-effects. In the past, this aspect of herbal medicines has made orthodox doctors rather sceptical as to whether any of them had any genuine benefits! There are one or two cautions that must be considered, however. If you experience problems with either remedy, stop taking them and you should have no further trouble.

It was mentioned in chapter 1 that the outer coat of the seed of the ginkgo could provoke an allergic reaction on the skin, causing raised welts such as those seen in nettle rash. It is best not to handle this part of the seed.

The medicinal part of ginkgo is the leaf. There have been no toxic effects revealed by clinical trials, with doses of up to 600mg a day, in one dose, of the standardised extract prepared from the leaf. Interestingly enough, in some trials the minor problems that people reported occurred as frequently in those taking the placebo as in those taking the true ginkgo. There is no evidence of toxicity at normal therapeutic doses. The problems that a few people have experienced whilst taking it have been limited to some degree of irritation of the digestive tract, which cleared up when they stopped taking ginkgo. A very few had headaches or other allergic reactions. There are no known drugs that ginkgo interacts with, though **if you are already taking medication from your doctor for circulatory problems, you should seek advice before starting either garlic or ginkgo.** One case has been recorded of an episode of bleeding in a person who was taking both ginkgo and aspirin, and a possible individual susceptibility to this must be considered by your doctor. The specific use of ginkgo during pregnancy has not been investigated and so, as with all medication that has not been specifically cleared for use during pregnancy, it is advisable not to try it in this situation.

Garlic is also considered clinically to be safe and non-toxic. The great majority of people who take it, for medical or culinary purposes, in amounts up to three times the recommended dose, have no problems at all with it. However, the raw clove contains some slightly acrid constituents that could cause discomfort to the digestive tract, with nausea, vomiting or diarrhoea in a few cases. The more likely problems are much milder, consisting of the characteristic symptoms of wind or 'repeating'. Some people have a more specific allergic reaction, and they will have to avoid the remedy.

The fresh juice, if it gets onto the skin, has been reported to cause irritation symptoms in some people. These are at worst a temporary problem: the skin should recover soon with no further problems. The fresh juice should not be used on skin that is broken or already inflamed, as this is more likely to cause irritation.

A potential interaction between garlic and the anticoagulant drug warfarin has been suggested, so, as with ginkgo, **if you are already taking medication for circulation problems or diabetes, check with your doctor before starting anything else**. Although there is no evidence of harmful effects during pregnancy, garlic has the traditional reputation of a plant that affects menstruation and pregnancy, so amounts greater than those commonly used in cooking are not advised during pregnancy.

A rather different matter is whether or not there are any health problems in which ginkgo and garlic should *not* be taken—that is, are they likely to aggravate anything? Advice from my colleagues suggests that the only condition they could aggravate is women's menopausal hot flushes. This is because during a hot flush much more blood than usual flows to the skin, so that heat can be lost from the skin to the air—this is the body's self-cooling mechanism. So of course anything that increases even further the flow of blood to the skin will result in more intensive feelings of flushing. Although hot flushes are in no way a dangerous problem, they are very uncomfortable and women who take ginkgo and garlic whilst they are going through the menopause should be aware of the possible aggravation.

CHAPTER 8

People's Experiences of Ginkgo

Case histories are about real people's actual experiences, rather than a scientific assessment of the efficacy of a particular medication on unknown 'standard' patients. Most people will have acquaintances who take garlic, and confirm its efficacy. The following accounts give an idea of some people's experiences of the less well known ginkgo.

Rosalind was a busy mother of three teenage boys, and holding down a very demanding job in personnel work, when she started to suffer from Ménière's disease. Her mother had suffered from the same problem, so there was an inherited tendency to it, and in the previous year her job had demanded long hours and difficult negotiations over staff redundancies. The first symptoms were a day of nausea and dizziness, and noises in the head which at the time Rosalind thought were due to food poisoning. She recovered and thought no more of it, until a second attack happened two weeks later. She thought perhaps she was using the VDU at work too much. Two months later she had an attack that was so severe she was vomiting, and unable to talk properly, slurring her speech. This happened again, so after a total of four months she visited her doctor. He diagnosed Ménière's disease, caused by a disturbance in the organ of balance in the inner ear. She was given some medication called Serc, which is the standard treatment for the condition. This suppressed the worst of the symptoms, but she still felt dizzy and nauseous most of the time. Three months later hospital tests confirmed the diagnosis, and she increased her medication by half as much again. There was no improvement.

Throughout the following year the best that she felt was dizzy, with the noises in her head becoming permanent. The worst was attacks so bad that they caused pain in her ears, total loss of balance, and vomiting. Rosalind had to carry a card saying that she was not drunk, but a sufferer from Ménière's disease, in case she suddenly fell over whilst out in public. She couldn't drive her car any more, and was dependent on her husband and sons (who were all very worried about her, and didn't like her to go out of their sight) for help with all the usual out-of-house activities that she had previously done by herself. Not surprisingly, her self-confidence dropped immensely, but she decided she was not going to give in to the illness, and continued to do her job. Sometimes she would have to go and lie down in a quiet, dark room at work for a while to cope with the bad attacks, but through the whole three and a half years of the illness, she took only a few days off work.

During that year her medication was increased to double and then treble the original amount, but with no improvement in symptoms. In the autumn there was one attack that lasted eleven hours, so bad that Rosalind couldn't speak or move, felt cold, clammy, was sweating and had pins and needles in both arms, and was hyperventilating. Two weeks later she was prescribed antihistamines as well as the Serc tablets, but the problems continued as before. The antihistamines were stopped and the Serc increased again, to four times the original dose.

In desperation, Rosalind agreed to have an operation on her ear. This was a sacrum decompression, and because of it she lost most of the hearing in that ear. Her lowest point came when she realised a month later that the attacks were just as bad, and she still had to continue the medication. The summer seemed to go better, but by the autumn she was back to the usual pattern of severe attacks. She decided to look for alternative treatments herself, and saw in a Midlands newspaper an article about a clinical trial to be carried out on ginkgo. It was appealing for sufferers from vertigo and tinnitus to volunteer to take part in this. Rosalind was so desperate that she felt she could not take the chance of volunteering and being turned down, so she decided to do her own trial by just buying ginkgo and taking it for a few months.

Having no guidance on the amount to take, she started off with 520mg a day (this is a much larger dose than that used in most clinical trials, but it caused no problems whatsoever). On the first day of taking it she started to feel better, and rapidly improved over the next two weeks. She has had no problems since, and has been taking the ginkgo for three months now. She has reduced the dosage to 240mg a day. In her own words:

'I feel as if I have my life back again. I am enjoying my job once more, and am driving my car. I can go out without worrying about collapsing in the street with an attack. If only I had known about this earlier—maybe the operation would have been unnecessary, with the result that my hearing would not have been so badly damaged and I would not have lost nearly four years of my life. I now feel immensely grateful that I did find *Ginkgo biloba*, and if I can share this knowledge with anyone else I am more than happy.'

*   *   *

The second account concerns a friend of mine called Andrew. For two years he suffered from a cough, trying many natural remedies without success. The cough wasn't due to an infection, but to irritation that had been caused by accidentally inhaling the dust from dried lavender flowers. The sensation Andrew got in his chest was an irritating tickle, which then provoked a bout of coughing, but there was no phlegm to be cleared from his chest. This suggested that there must have been some residual inflammation in his airways long after the lavender dust would have been engulfed in mucus and cleared out. In fact, he had a sense of muscle spasm in his chest, like a weight there, but not the constriction or wheezing associated with asthma. As luck would have it, he tried taking ginkgo for a completely different problem, and noticed one week after he started it that the cough had gone. He took it for three weeks in total, which proved to be enough to prevent the cough returning. His advice is that ginkgo is worth trying if you have a dry, irritating cough (so long as the cause is not connected with an infection—you would need garlic as well in that case).

* * *

We now come to circulation problems. Plenty of people with a tendency to feel the cold badly in the winter have benefited from taking ginkgo for this. All those I know of have been elderly people, and I think it likely, therefore, that they would all have some degree of deterioration in the condition of their blood vessels: ginkgo may well be helping them to reduce the consequences of this. So it can't be guaranteed that a younger person, who feels the cold as a constitutional tendency but does not have any great deterioration in the condition of the circulation, would get the same benefit—the basic problem that ginkgo puts right would not be present in such a case.

Another aspect of circulatory problems is the tendency to feel too hot, especially in the feet. This happened to Caroline, a friend of mine in her early sixties, and was very troublesome in hot weather. Her doctor diagnosed it as a condition known as Raynaud's syndrome. It is caused by a temporary constriction in the small arteries of the hands and feet, usually brought on by exposure to the cold. It can also be associated with blockage to the flow of blood in arteries between the wrist and forearm. Caroline contacted a self-help group for Raynaud's sufferers, and saw in their literature that ginkgo was a suggested treatment. Like Rosalind, she had no guidance as to the dosage and started by taking 750mg a day with no problems. The burning feelings calmed down and have since happened only very occasionally in the summer. Caroline has been taking ginkgo for four years now, and has reduced the dose to 250mg daily. Although the burning troubles her very little, she intends to continue with ginkgo for its protective action on the circulation and brain.

* * *

In the next case both the preventative and curative properties are important. Alice, aged forty-four, is one of my patients and has become a very good friend. Over the six years she has consulted me, her problems have revolved around the stress she experiences in her work as a civil servant, in various management roles. This has led to headaches, blood pressure hovering around the marginally high range, and may well have aggravated the psoriasis she has suffered from since she was eight years old. She tends to have fluid retention in her ankles, which is aggravated by hot weather. As well as a busy job, she is currently taking a course of further study, causing more time pressures.

Although she knows about the need for a good diet, food is a lower priority to her than other commitments, so that our discussions about the right food to keep her healthy usually have only a temporary effect. Exercise is another factor which gets a low priority in her busy life. Cigarettes have been a long-term habit which Alice admits is unlikely to change. Over the years whilst she has been taking my medicine I have managed most of the time to help her cope with the stress of her work, the headaches and the psoriasis (though this fluctuates). When I was researching this book, it occurred to me that, in view of her smoking and marginally high blood pressure, ginkgo would be an excellent remedy for her to take long term for the protective action it would have on her circulation. I also hoped for an improvement in the psoriasis which, as usual, was getting worse with the return of the colder weather in autumn.

Alice has been taking ginkgo for about four months now. Over the winter she says that she has felt the cold less severely than in previous years, and despite the usual amount of stress, the psoriasis is better than she can ever remember it being at this time of year (late winter). She needs to take it for longer to be more conclusive about the benefits, and considering that it is intended to ameliorate the harmful consequences of smoking and highish blood pressure, it will be very difficult to assess its effect as we shall not know what problems would develop if she were not taking it. I can say, though, that so long as she is taking it I feel much happier about her chances of maintaining a healthy circulation into her later years, to enable her to keep up her busy way of life.

* * *

You might think these accounts of ginkgo persuasive enough to justify its acceptance as a valid treatment. Scientists, however, would judge these histories to be merely anecdotal evidence, and this is not enough to gain recognition for its benefits. This is because, in any group of people, responses to any type of treatment will vary, just as most of their other characteristics show variation. Shape, size, tastes in food, energy levels, eye colour—we are all completely individual, with many factors influencing our health. With any medical treatment, some people will show no response to it, some will have a dramatic response, and most will fall somewhere in between these extremes. If we base our assessment of the efficacy of a remedy on only a few cases, we don't know whether they are showing a typical response, or an extreme one. So we can't use this as a basis to predict whether someone else suffering from cardiovascular disease can expect the same benefit from trying ginkgo and garlic. In case histories it is the individual that is important, but clinical trials give a different type of information. In trials, it is the overall results shown by a number of otherwise unknown people that count. The trials provide objective evidence to support the theories on the uses of medicines. And there are plenty of trials on both ginkgo and garlic, a fact which reflects the size of the problem that heart disease and asthma pose to the Western world.

The setting up of a convincing clinical trial is a difficult matter. First of all the researchers have to decide exactly what they want to test for. They then have to find suitable people who agree to take part. It is necessary to find participants whose health problems are very similar, so that the results obtained at the end are clear to understand. There will always be a range of responses to the treatment that need to be carefully interpreted. And there must be a certain number of participants in the trial who are not given the substance under test, but who don't know this. They are given an inert *placebo*, and their improvement must be noted and compared with that of the group which was given the real substance, called the *verum*. (A number of people will always improve in the placebo group, even though they have not received any active medication. This phenomenon is called the *placebo effect*. The improvement in the verum group must be significantly greater than that shown by the placebo group if the therapy is to be accepted as effective.) The trial must be designed and carried out in such a way that there is no doubt or ambiguity about the interpretation of the results. Many trials are considered invalid on this basis, and the results will not be accepted. Such trials of new medicines, whether derived from natural sources or from industrial processes, are taking place continuously. They are designed to show that the medicines are both safe and effective, and only after this is a new treatment allowed a product licence for manufacture and sale.

Some trials are carried out by drugs companies looking for new products. Some are carried out in research institutions. Plenty of trials have taken place on both ginkgo and garlic in the last twenty years. Some have been judged to be inconclusive but many have been accepted as valid. If you are interested in the results of these, you will find them described in Part Two of the book.

CHAPTER 9

The Clinical Actions of Ginkgo and Garlic

Clinical trials have shown quite conclusively that both ginkgo and garlic are valid therapeutic agents which are effective in the treatment of a variety of conditions and diseases. This chapter looks in more detail at the areas of confirmed therapeutic action and, backed by current research, suggests possible mechanisms which might explain the actions of ginkgo and garlic.

The ancestry of garlic is botanically very distant from that of ginkgo; they are not even in the same class of plants, garlic being a member of the class *angiospermae* and ginkgo belonging to the more ancient class of *gymnospermae*. As one might expect, the two plants are also biochemically very dissimilar with regard to their therapeutic constituents, garlic producing disulphide compounds and ginkgo terpenes (ginkgolides) and phenolics. It is rather strange, therefore, or at least something of a coincidence, to find that not only do garlic and ginkgo prove to be effective in treating the same range of cardiovascular diseases, but also the therapeutic mechanism of their actions shows remarkable similarities at a biochemical and cellular level. Table 1 summarises the actions of garlic and ginkgo and relates these actions to their therapeutic applications.

Table 1   Summary of the main actions and therapeutic uses of ginkgo and garlic

Plant	Actions [reference]	therapeutic applications
GARLIC	inhibition of platelet aggregation and adhesion [5][6][14][21]	asthma arterial disease
	free radical scavenger [35]	cerebral and other ischaemias arterial disease
	inhibits LDL oxidation and production of free radicals [19]	cerebral and other ischaemias arterial disease
	inhibition of arachidonic acid metabolism [41]	asthma arterial disease
	reduces plasma LDL levels [1][4][8][31][38][44][50]	arterial disease
	reduction in blood viscosity [14]	arterial disease
	antimicrobial [29]	bacterial infections
GINKGO	inhibition of platelet aggregation and adhesion [44]	asthma arterial disease
	free radical scavenger [32][25]	cerebral and other ischaemias
	inhibition of PAF [12][44]	asthma arterial disease

Looking at the table it can be seen that many of the actions of ginkgo and garlic are haematological in nature, closely connected with platelets and the biochemistry of the interactions between platelets and other associated cells. Over the past few years there has been much research on the role of platelets and their relationship with cardiovascular and respiratory disorders.[34][18] In this chapter we shall, firstly, briefly examine the normal functioning of platelets in the clotting process, then consider their role in the pathology of various diseases and finally look at how ginkgo and garlic act as therapeutic agents within the context of that pathology.

Platelets and the clotting process

Platelets, or *thrombocytes* to give them their scientific name, are small, non-nucleated, disc-shaped cell fragments, 3–4µm diameter, that circulate in the blood. There are around 300 million in each millilitre of blood and they have an effective life of around ten days. They are produced by a budding off process from large cells called *megakaryocytes*, which are found primarily in the bone marrow and also in the lungs. Platelets are co-mediators in the clotting function that is normally a response to vascular damage and, together with various other cells, chemicals and plasma proteins, they provide an effective means of inhibiting haemorrhage.

Platelets normally circulate in the blood, inactive unless they are in the proximity of an area of tissue damage. In this case the platelets are likely to encounter *collagen*, a protein found in the connective tissue under the blood vessel endothelium that normally isolates the collagen from the circulating platelets. In the damaged blood vessel wall, platelets will come into contact with collagen that will activate them, causing them to swell, become more sticky, and trigger the same process in other platelets until they clump together to form a plug. Other chemicals associated with tissue damage are able to activate platelets and these include *thrombin*, *PAF*, (platelet activating factor), *adrenaline* (epinephrine) and *ADP* (adenosine diphosphate). These substances are termed *agonists*. This clumping together of the platelets causes them to become activated and start to release *thromboxane* and more PAF, both of which act as *vasoconstrictors*. The smooth muscle surrounding the blood vessel contracts and restricts the flow of blood, so preventing haemorrhage. Other chemicals that are released encourage other platelets to adhere to the original platelets and this forms a *platelet plug*. To assist in the repair of the damage, platelets release *PDGF* (platelet derived growth factor) which acts as a signal for smooth muscle cells surrounding the damaged vessel to multiply and also

93

for *fibroblasts* to lay down new extra cellular matrix. PDGF also acts as a chemoattractant to fibroblasts and macrophages, the latter helping to prevent bacterial infection of the wound. If the area of damage is very small this plug may be enough to prevent blood loss, and the tiny injuries that happen every day as we bump into chairs, tables and doors are repaired in the manner outlined above. Figure 6 outlines how platelets respond to damage of the vascular wall.

If the injury is severe a *blood clot* will form, triggered by chemicals released from the platelets and the damaged vessel wall. These cause soluble blood proteins to transform into insoluble threads called *fibrin*, which form a tangled mass that enmeshes passing red blood cells. You can see the effects of this process in any minor skin wound where the bleeding stops after a few minutes. Any deficiency in the substances that are involved in clot formation is a serious problem, as in the case of haemophilia. On the other hand, problems causing an increased tendency towards clotting (hypercoagulation) are just as dangerous and very common.

The mechanism of clotting is, as you may guess, quite complex, involving a cascade of clotting factors, few of which have particularly memorable names. There are two pathways that can initiate clotting, the *extrinsic* pathway that involves chemicals released from damaged cells outside the blood vessels, and the *intrinsic* pathway caused by platelets activated by collagen exposure within the blood vessels. Both pathways lead to the formation of the enzyme *prothrombinase* which converts *prothrombin* to *thrombin* which in turn converts the soluble plasma protein *fibrinogen* to the insoluble fibrin threads that, with blood cells, create the clot. The fibrin matrix is further stabilised by *Fibrin Stabilising Factor XIII*. Figure 7 shows an outline of the intrinsic and extrinsic pathways.

It is the intrinsic pathway that may be a significant factor in cases of chronic vascular disease because the formation of atherosclerotic plaques specifically causes the exposure of collagen and thus the initiation of the clotting process.

The main factor that prevents the initiation of the clotting process in normal, undamaged vessels is the smooth surface of the cells lining the blood vessels—the endothelium. Also, certain chemicals

94

Figure 6   The activation and action of platelets in response to damage of the vascular endothelium

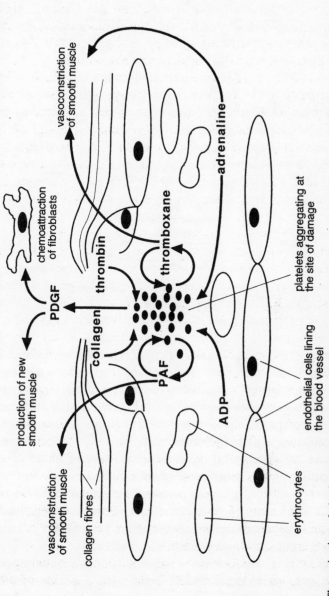

The activation of platelets to form a platelet plug by exposed collagen and newly formed thrombin. Platelets themselves produce PAF and thromboxane which stimulate other platelets to aggregate and produce PAF and thromboxane. Both of these chemicals, along with adrenaline, are vasoconstrictors which reduce the blood flow in the damaged vessel. PDGF (platelet derived growth factor) starts repair by causing smooth muscle cells to divide and attract fibroblasts which produce new collagen.

Figure 7   The intrinsic and extrinsic clotting pathways

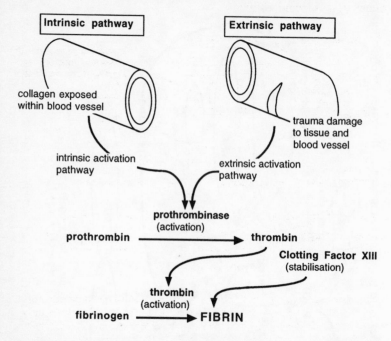

including *prostacyclin* and *EDNO* (endothelium derived nitric oxide), produced in the endothelial cells, oppose the clotting processes and are effective unless there is a great increase in the clot-promoting chemicals, mentioned above, which are produced when damage occurs. The relationship between platelets and the endothelium is extremely complicated and there is good evidence that the maintenance of the endothelial lining of blood vessels is dependent on the presence of platelets in the blood. Sufferers of *thrombocytopaenia* (lack of platelets) have been shown to exhibit a lack of integrity of the endothelium which is reversed when the platelet numbers return to normal. Figure 8 details the relationship between the intact endothelium and platelets.

As we have seen above, the activation of platelets in response to damage to the endothelium of blood vessels is a very complicated process (and the processes here have been simplified considerably).

Figure 8   Inhibition of platelet adhesion and aggregation by the intact vascular endothelium

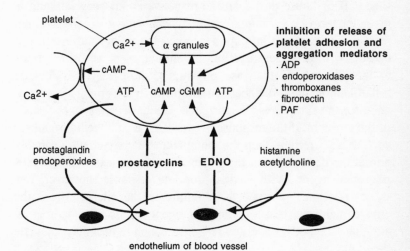

endothelium of blood vessel

In the undamaged endothelium, various factors mediate in the prevention of platelet adhesion and aggregation. Histamine and acetylcholine promote the release of prostacyclins and EDNO (endothelium derived nitric oxide) which cause the platelet to produce cAMP and cGMP. These reduce intracellular levels of Ca^{2+} by sequestering Ca^{2+} in the α granules and inhibiting the uptake of Ca^{2+} from extracellular sources. The α granules are thus inhibited from releasing their platelet adhesion and aggregation mediators. The role of prostaglandin endoperoxides released from platelets is uncertain in the relationship between platelets and the endothelium.

Where there is such a complex interchange of messages and materials there is always the possibility of malfunction, and it is now recognised that the inappropriate activation of platelets can produce, or at least contribute to, many of the pathologies associated with disorders of the circulatory and respiratory systems.

Asthma
At the heart of an asthma attack is the allergen response, also known as the anaphylactic response, a complex series of immunological reactions to a pathogenic or toxic substance. If the allergen

is a dangerous pathogenic organism then the response is justified and necessary, but if it is caused by a household pet, a common foodstuff or house dust then the response is inappropriate and is given the term *Type 1 anaphylactic hypersensitivity*. In the allergen response, the discomfort experienced by the asthma sufferer is not caused by the allergen itself but by the body's powerful reactions to the allergen. In the case of asthma, these reactions include inflammation and bronchoconstriction which are primarily responsible for the symptoms. Treating the patient depends on the cause of the problem. If the response is caused by a pathogenic organism such as a bacterium, then the therapeutic strategy would probably aim at the destruction of the organism with, for example, an antimicrobial agent. With an inappropriate response, however, this is not possible, so apart from removing the allergen from the environment, the best a therapeutic agent can do is to dampen or attenuate the body's allergen response which in turn may alleviate the symptoms.

The pathology of asthma is extremely complex, as is any immune response, and the sequence of events leading to an asthma attack is not fully understood—certainly not at the cellular and biochemical levels. The traditional model of an interaction between antigens and mast cells in the lung epithelium has been subject to much revision over the past few years as research has revealed more about the chemical interactions that occur between different types of cells to produce the anaphylactic attack. There is much debate amongst research scientists regarding the contribution of various mediators such as histamines, thromboxanes, platelet activating factor, leukotrienes and so on to bronchospasm and inflammation, but there is general agreement on one precept, namely that there is no one mediator that is responsible for asthma.

Recently, much attention has been focused on the role of platelets in asthma or, more precisely, on one of the activators of platelets, platelet activating factor or PAF [18][27]. No one is quite sure of the exact role of platelets in asthma, but research is increasingly demonstrating that a connection does exist. Platelets are produced by megakaryocytes that are found in great numbers in the bone marrow and it is generally assumed that this is the main site of platelet production. Recently, however, it has been observed that abnormal numbers of megakaryocytes are found in the pulmonary arteries of asthmatics and it has been speculated that in these cases platelet production may also take place in the lungs. Certainly, platelets are found in increasing numbers in the lungs of asthmatics, but this has been shown to be due mainly to the aggregating action of PAF rather than just coincidental as a place of production. Levels of PAF have also shown to be elevated in asthmatics concomitant with a decrease in levels of serum *PAF acetylhydrolase*, the enzyme that inactivates PAF [46]. Platelets have been shown to have IgE receptors on their surface membranes, allowing them to respond directly to antigen and perhaps triggering the anaphylactic response by the release of thromboxane, PAF and other mediators.

Eosinophils are also appearing more often in research papers as correspondents in the platelet and asthma link. These large polymorphonuclear leucocytes are associated with allergic responses. Platelet activating factor (PAF) is a strong chemoattractant for eosinophils that themselves have the ability to produce large quantities of PAF, and this positive feedback mechanism has been postulated as a possible mechanism for the progressive increase in symptoms during an asthma attack. Also, the eosinophils found in asthmatic patients appear to be sensitised, as they demonstrate a faster response to substances such as PAF released during allergic inflammation [47]. Platelets are also able to activate eosinophils to perform their cytotoxic function, producing *ECP* (eosinophil cationic protein) and *EDN* (eosinophil derived neurotoxin), and these have been implicated in damage to the epithelial and neurological tissue common in asthma.

Mast cells are also an important link in the anaphylactic response. Found within the lung epithelium, they respond to allergens and release a complex suite of mediators by various pathways; amongst these are histamine, PAF, leukotrienes, prostaglandins and thromboxanes which between them are responsible for the inflammation, bronchoconstriction and vasodilation that are typical pathophysiological reactions in asthma.

Platelet activating factor, produced by platelets, eosinophils and mast cells, is now considered to possess many of the characteristics that identify it as one of the central mediators in the anaphylactic response. Tests have shown that it is a potent mediator of bronchoconstriction, vascular permeability and sustained inflammation, three conditions typical of the pathology of asthma. A summary of the putative relationships between platelets and other cells involved in asthma is shown in Figure 9.

The effect of ginkgo and garlic on these processes is still to be determined. Research has demonstrated that ginkgo does attenuate the anaphylactic response, and undoubtedly this effect is in a major part due to ginkgolide B that is known to be a potent *PAF antagonist*. Both garlic and ginkgo have also been shown to prevent platelet aggregation, a process that releases even more PAF. The mechanism of PAF antagonism by ginkgo is presumed to be by the blocking of receptors on the platelet membrane. Garlic has been shown to have the ability to inhibit the metabolism of arachidonic acid that is a precursor of both the cyclo-oxygenase and lipoxygenase pathways. In the case of asthma this would be of therapeutic benefit as it should, in theory, contribute to a reduction in the release of leukotrienes, prostaglandins and thromboxanes and so attenuate the bronchoconstriction, inflammation and oedema, characteristic of an asthma attack.

Platelet activating factor produced by degranulation of mast cells has a stimulatory effect on the activation of platelets and eosinophils and their release of even larger quantities of PAF. The inhibition of PAF by ginkgolide B could be reasonably expected to attenuate the eosinophil response. This could in turn reduce the amount of damage to the airway epithelium by the cytotoxic products released by the eosinophils.

More clinical research needs to be done to assess the effect of ginkgo and garlic on asthma. Traditionally, both have been used to treat pulmonary disorders, and case histories indicate that this treatment has been successful. Unfortunately, the aetiology of the disorders described in some of these case histories is not always clear so it would be rather presumptuous to claim sound, empirical evi-

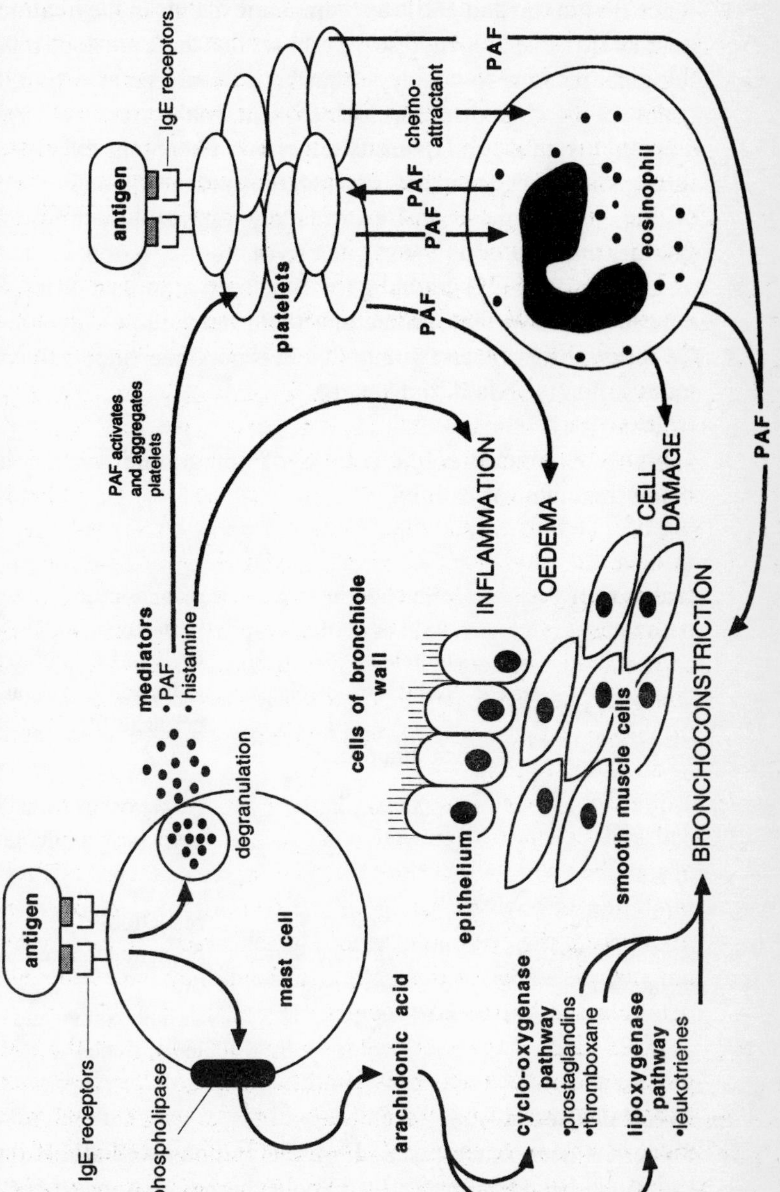

Figure 9 Proposed relationship between platelets and other cells in the lung involved in asthma

dence for ginkgo and garlic as therapeutic agents in the treatment of asthma. However, recent research shows that there are good pharmacological reasons to conclude that both should be effective in the treatment of this disorder and clinical trials are now urgently required to qualify and quantify the effect. There may even be some synergistic effect if they are used together and there is some evidence that this may be the case. Unfortunately, asthma is such a complex disorder that one would be suspicious of the suggestion that any one (or even two) agents could be totally effective in its control. However, given the variable nature of asthma and the sound evidence for the actions of garlic and ginkgo, there is good reason to believe that some sufferers should find benefit.

Table 2   Summary of the actions of ginkgo and garlic relevant to the treatment of asthma

action	result	physiological effect
inhibition of PAF	reduction in the activation of platelets reduction in release of PAF and thromboxane	reduction of bronchoconstriction by PAF and thromboxanes reduction in vascular permeability (oedema)
	reduction in the activation of eosinophils	reduction in damage to bronchial epithelium
inhibition of arachidonic acid metabolism	inhibition of lipoxygenase and cyclo-oxygenase pathways	reduction in bronchoconstriction by prostaglandins, thromboxanes and leukotrienes

Arterial disease

There has been much research on the pathology of atherogenesis, and much has been discovered about the interactions of cells and chemicals associated with the disease, but there is no unified theory that satisfactorily explains all aspects of the process. It is of no surprise, therefore, that the precise role of platelets and their associated mediators in the pathology of atherogenesis is not fully understood although there is general agreement amongst researchers that they are important factors in the process. The formation of thrombi (thrombogenesis), often associated with atherosclerosis, indisputably involves platelets, but again, whether they are a causative agent in the formation of the thrombi or just one of many participants in their formation is a question yet to be fully answered. In either case, though, the thrombus is an inappropriate manifestation of the clotting process and we know that the activation of platelets is important in this process [34].

Early in the life of some individuals, the first recognisable event in the development of atherosclerotic plaques is the formation of fatty streaks under the endothelium of the arteries. The causal factors in the transformation of these streaks into atherosclerotic plaques probably involves an interaction of chemical, dietary and immune agents. Viral damage has also been implicated, particularly cytomegalovirus. Macrophages called *foam cells*, laden with fat droplets of LDL (low density lipoprotein), migrate to the subendothelium and some smooth muscle cells also appear to be transformed into these foam cells. The endothelium also appears to become more permeable to LDL, contributing to the build-up of lipids in the subendothelium. The LDL reacts with oxidative mediators secreted by the endothelium, which causes oxidation of the lipids, the production of free radicals and the release of chemoattractants that promote the migration of more macrophages to the area, so increasing the size of the lesion [26][42].

These factors may cause damage to the cells and connective tissue of the endothelial lining of the arteries, which in turn triggers the body's repair mechanisms. Platelets arriving at the damaged area release *PDGF* (platelet derived growth factor), and *mitogen* (a substance that promotes mitosis), and this initiates the proliferation of the smooth muscle cells that surround the artery. Macrophages also release PDGF which exacerbates the problem. The smooth muscle cells secrete collagen, elastin and glycoproteins, causing the fatty streaks to enlarge and become more fibrous in nature. The fatty streak has become an atherosclerotic plaque, being fibrous and rich in lipids.

The initiation of this process and its progressive development may be dependent on genetic and environmental factors (diet, smoking and exercise, etc.), not to mention disease factors such as hypertension and hypercholesterolaemia. Some of these are discussed elsewhere in this book. Some plaques may remain relatively small, whilst others enlarge to the point of occluding the artery, causing ischaemia and conditions such as angina pectoris.

Damage to the endothelial cells caused by various mediators in the development of the plaque can initiate events leading to the formation of a thrombus, a process called *thrombogenesis*. Inflammatory events around the plaque such as ulceration can expose the subendothelium of the artery and the collagen fibres contained in it. Platelets have a strong affinity for collagen and exposure to it triggers a cascade of clotting events described at the beginning of this chapter. These involve PAF and thromboxane, both strong platelet aggregating and adhesion mediators released by the platelets themselves. Exposed collagen also triggers the intrinsic pathway that results in thrombin, another potent platelet aggregation factor, and fibrin, which produces the insoluble matrix of the clot. As with the formation of atheromas, the progression of thrombogenesis depends on genetic predisposition and disease states such as an increased tendency of the blood to coagulate (hypercoagulability), often associated with venous thrombosis and pulmonary embolism.

The development of arterial disease is not solely a one-way process, and it progresses against the actions of the body's own repair mechanisms that attempt to repair damaged tissue and remove inappropriate clots. In many cases these are adequate to keep arterial diseases in check, so in many of the cases where the disease state prevails, it is undoubtedly due to shortcomings in these repair mechanisms rather than the hyperactivation of damage mediators. This concept is important when developing any therapeutic regime that should, if possible, support existing mechanisms for the resolution of the disease.

Figure 10 Development of an atherosclerotic plaque and thrombus

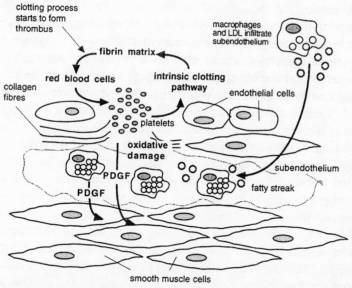

The events in the arterial wall associated with the development of an atheromatous plaque and thrombus. Macrophages and LDL invade the subendothelium where oxidation of the lipids causes damage to the endothelial lining, exposing collagen fibres which in turn attract platelets. PDGF (platelet derived growth factor) causes the smooth muscle cells to proliferate and increase the size of the plaque. Platelets release chemicals that initiate the clotting process and initiate the formation of a thrombus.

Figure 10 depicts some of the events leading to the formation of an atheromatous plaque and associated thrombus.

With such a complex disease, treatment must take into account the aetiology of the problem. Certain anticoagulatory drugs have been found to decrease the incidence of thromboembolism by their anticoagulatory effects. Aspirin has proved to be an effective therapeutic agent, although its effect on the gastric mucosa means that it is not suitable for everyone. There is considerable evidence *in vivo* and *in vitro* that garlic and ginkgo (neither of which has clinical side-effects) can both be very useful in the treatment of atheroma and thrombi.

The regular ingestion of raw garlic is undoubtedly of great therapeutic benefit to individuals at risk from atherosclerosis and thrombosis, and it acts directly against factors evident in the formation of plaques and thrombi. There are also some actions of ginkgo that would recommend it as an anti-atherosclerotic agent.

Firstly, there is evidence that garlic reinforces the processes that maintain the endothelial lining of the normal blood vessel by inhibiting platelet adhesion and aggregation. The activation of both prostacyclins and EDNO (endothelium derived nitric oxide) has been observed to be promoted by garlic [5][13]. Both of these substances inhibit the release of platelet derived adhesion and aggregation mediators such as thromboxanes and PAF.

Secondly, garlic has been shown to reduce those factors in the blood predisposing the individual to atherosclerosis. In numerous trials, the plasma levels of LDL have been shown to be significantly reduced by garlic and this should in turn reduce the LDL uptake by macrophages associated with the formation of the plaques [1][4][8][31][43][49]. Garlic has been shown to reduce the viscosity of the blood that is linked to its propensity to coagulate and form thrombi. Serum fibrinogen levels have also been shown to be significantly reduced by garlic, which should again reduce the coagulability of the blood [14].

Thirdly, recent research has shown that garlic actively inhibits the formation of atherosclerotic plaques. Studies on the atherosclerotic plaques of human aorta *in vitro* have shown that garlic reduces the level of cholesteryl esters and free cholesterol in the plaques, but there is little evidence of the mechanism that achieves this effect [33]. Garlic extract has been shown to inhibit the oxidative modification of LDL, which in consequence will reduce free radical damage [19]. Both garlic and ginkgo have also been shown to be strong free radical scavengers [36][40].

Fourthly, it has been demonstrated that both garlic and ginkgo, especially the latter, are potent antagonists for PAF (platelet activating factor), one of the key chemicals in platelet aggregation and the formation of clots or thrombi [25][40]. Raw garlic also inhibits arachidonic acid metabolism as well as dose-dependent inhibition of cyclo-oxygenase activity [2][5][41]. Arachidonic acid metabolites feed into the cyclo-oxygenase pathway, resulting in the formation of various mediators, including thromboxanes, which are potent platelet activating chemicals. Any inhibition of this pathway could assist the natural anticoagulatory factors to resist the formation of inappropriate clots.

Table 3   Summary of the actions of garlic and ginkgo relevant to the treatment of arterial disease

action	result	physiological effect
GARLIC		
activation of prostacyclins and EDNO (endothelium derived nitric oxide)	inhibits platelet release of ADP, thromboxanes, fibronectin and PAF	inhibits platelet adhesion and aggregation so maintaining normal endothelium
reduces plasma LDL levels	reduces uptake of LDL by macrophages	reduces rate of plaque growth
reduces viscocity of blood and serum fibrinogen levels	reduces tendency of blood to clot	reduces rate of thrombus growth
reduces uptake of cholesterol into subendothelium	reduces levels of free cholesterol in plaques	reduces rate of plaque growth
inhibits LDL oxidation	inhibits production of free radicals	reduces cell damage by free radicals so inhibiting atherogenesis
free radical scavenger	reduces levels of free radicals	reduces cell damage by free radicals so inhibiting atherogenesis
PAF antagonist	inhibits platelet adhesion and aggregation and release of mediators	inhibits formation of thrombi

107

Table 3 *continued.*

inhibits arachidonic acid metabolism	reduces cyclo-oxygenase activity and production of thromboxanes	inhibits formation of thrombi
GINKGO free radical scavenger	reduces levels of free radicals	reduces cell damage by free radicals so inhibiting atherogenesis
PAF antagonist	inhibits platelet adhesion and aggregation and release of mediators	inhibits formation of thrombi

There seems to be good evidence for a difference in efficacy between fresh garlic and dried garlic presented in powdered form. Several researchers have commented on this and undoubtedly the use of processed garlic has contributed to the negative results produced in a small minority of studies [2][38].

Hypertension

Hypertension is usually diagnosed where an individual presents a systolic pressure above 150mm Hg and a diastolic pressure of above 95mm Hg. However, diagnosis of hypertension is probably the easiest part of the treatment of this problematical disorder. In 90 per cent of cases, the cause of high blood pressure is unknown (called primary or idiopathic hypertension). Treatment will therefore proceed against the symptoms rather than the underlying cause. Hypertension often accelerates the process of atherosclerosis that further occludes the arteries, so worsening the problem of hypertension. Treatment usually includes diuretics and the dietary restriction of salt, both of which decrease the plasma volume, together with vasodilators to decrease peripheral resistance. Exercise and weight reduction in cases of obesity have also been shown to help. Clinical trials have demonstrated that garlic can help in mild cases of hypertension [8][37] and its ability to reduce the viscocity of the blood would perhaps explain its short-term action. Ginkgo has also been shown to reduce viscocity and improve peripheral circulation [24]. In the longer term, however, the effectiveness of garlic will depend on the aetiology of the problem—which in 90 per cent of cases will be unknown. Certainly, where atherosclerosis has been diagnosed along with hypertension, then both garlic and ginkgo will help arrest the progression of the disease, as described in detail above.

Cerebral insufficiency
Degenerative dementia may involve many complex changes within the brain tissue of the sufferer, including the degeneration of neurons and an impairment of neuronal transmission leading to memory loss and cognitive impairment. These may be related to an interference with the blood supply leading to insufficiency in oxygen and glucose, both of which are essential for normal neurological functions. These circumstances may cause transient ischaemia, a temporary shortage of blood, followed by a return of oxygenated blood (reperfusion) and it is the reperfusion that is believed to generate platelet activating factor (PAF). This alkyl-phospholipid is produced by many types of cell, including platelets and endothelial cells. PAF has been shown to increase during brain trauma and although its actions are not completely understood, it is believed that it may amplify the damage caused by excessive glutamate, released during trauma. Obviously, in these circumstances, any substance that will reduce the effect of PAF will have a beneficial effect and *Ginkgo biloba*, especially ginkgolide B of the terpene fraction, has been shown to be a strong PAF antagonist [12][40][44]. PAF has also been implicated in the generation of oxygenated metabolites of arachidonic acid and free superoxide radicals (0_2-.) which are highly reactive and destructive. *Ginkgo biloba* is a strong scavenger of superoxide free radicals [32], and reducing their number may have a significant protective effect.

Without further research, we can only speculate whether the above mechanisms accurately explain the neuroprotective action of ginkgo, but the evidence from numerous clinical trials has certainly demonstrated its effectiveness as a therapeutic agent in the treatment of cerebral ischaemia [10][15][22][36][48]. No doubt, as our understanding of the pathology of this disorder increases, so will our understanding of the mechanism whereby ginkgo exerts its beneficial effect.

Intermittent claudication

This is predominantly a disease of advancing years caused by occlusion of the arteries in the leg, due mainly to atherosclerotic lesions. It is often complicated by a reduction in competence of valves of the deep veins of the leg. This delays the efficient venous removal of blood from the lower limbs and the consequential emptying of blood from the capillary bed of the muscles. These conditions also predispose the individual to thrombosis and oedema.

The muscles in the lower limbs are the most metabolically active tissues, and consequently they are also those most likely to be affected by any inadequacy in the supply of blood. Any increase in physical activity, such as walking, increases the demand for energy to which the muscle cells respond by increasing their rate of cellular respiration. This increase in respiration requires more oxygen, and any impairment in the circulation due to atherosclerotic lesions can lead to semi-anaerobic conditions in some of the muscles; the lactic acid produced induces pain that is relieved only when the exercise stops and the supply of blood becomes sufficient for aerobic respiration again.

The strategy used in the treatment of arterial occlusive disease depends on the stage to which the disease has progressed. Early treatments may include drugs to halt the advance of atherosclerosis, including antiplatelet agents. Vasodilatory drugs, although in theory conferring some benefit, have instead been found to divert blood to other areas rather than improving the blood supply to the legs. Anticoagulatory drugs may help prevent the formation of thrombi. Physiotherapy has proved beneficial, as has vascular reconstruction in more severe cases.

Clinical trials have shown ginkgo to be of benefit to sufferers of intermittent claudication [9][28]. Ginkgo improves the supply of oxygenated blood, as demonstrated by transcutaneous oximetry, and it has also been shown to enhance the microcirculation in tissues and decrease the viscoelasticity of blood [24]. However, the precise method by which ginkgo exerts this effect is unclear.

The beneficial effects of garlic in the inhibition of the development and progression of arterial disease have already been discussed at some length (above). The antiplatelet action of garlic and its tendency to inhibit atherogenesis could prove an effective long-term strategy in the management of chronic arterial ischaemia. Naturally, this therapy should be used in conjunction with a carefully controlled exercise and dietary regime, together with immediate cessation of deleterious habits such as smoking which exacerbate the problem.

Deafness, tinnitus and Ménière's syndrome

Diseases associated with the eighth cranial nerve include deafness, tinnitus and Ménière's syndrome, all of which have been shown to respond to treatment with ginkgo [16][17][39] (see also chapter 8). The aetiologies of these disorders are varied; deafness has a variety of causes, as has tinnitus, but lesions of the sensory neurons in the internal ear are regularly a common feature. Ménière's syndrome is the result of a gross dilation of the endolymph system of the internal ear, resulting in further degenerative changes and often leading to deafness. Undoubtedly, ginkgo has some neuroprotective effect, possibly by inhibition of platelet activating factor and possibly in its role as a scavenger of free radicals, but any suggestion of the therapeutic mechanism would be speculative [40]. However, given the positive results from clinical trials and the absence of known side-effects, the treatment of these chronic disorders with ginkgo could be justified.

Premenstrual syndrome

This is a suite of conditions, characterised by emotional instability, irritability, general oedema and tenderness of the breasts, which occurs in the week before menstruation and disappears a few hours after its onset. PMS is undoubtedly due to the changing hormonal levels of oestrogen and progesterone prior to menstruation, but how these initiate many of the symptoms of PMS is uncertain. Certainly some of the symptoms suggest a relationship with the circulatory system, which is an area where both ginkgo and garlic are known to have an effect. However, it would be too speculative to propose any coherent hypothesis about the action of ginkgo and garlic on PMS until more is known about the condition. There have been relatively few trials of ginkgo in the treatment of PMS, but the most recent one by Tamborini and Taurelle [45] in France showed that ginkgo did help attenuate symptoms, both physical and neurophysiological. Congestive symptoms associated with the breasts were particularly improved.

CHAPTER 10

Clinical Trials of Ginkgo and Garlic

New pharmaceutical products are being developed and put on the market every day, but before these products are released for sale they need to be thoroughly tested in the laboratory to see whether the drug in question has any beneficial or detrimental effects. Ultimately, however, the new product must be tested on real patients in a carefully monitored clinical trial which will determine how it compares with other similar drugs and whether there are any side-effects.

Some new products are in fact quite old ones which have been in use for many years, sometimes for centuries, but until recently their effectiveness has never been tested scientifically; such is the case for many natural products of plant origin—for example, garlic and ginkgo. Even if the usefulness of these traditional remedies has been demonstrated by the positive results obtained in treatment, it may still be useful to quantify their benefit. Sometimes it is necessary to conduct clinical trials in order to demonstrate the usefulness of natural medicines to orthodox practitioners who demand hard data about their effectiveness. Sometimes, especially with chronic diseases, such as problems of the circulatory system and atherosclerosis, the effects of treatment with a particular remedy may not be apparent in the short term. This is because, although changes may be extremely beneficial, causing, for example, a decrease in serum cholesterol, they may not be easily detected in the consulting room. In these cases, a scientifically controlled clinical trial can provide useful information because equipment not normally found in the consulting

113

room can be used to measure small but significant changes in serum cholesterol in response to a particular remedy.

For any trial or study to have validity, certain parameters need to be satisfied, but primarily any trial should be fair and free from bias. The most commonly accepted method of ensuring that trials are fair is by making them *placebo-controlled* and *double-blind*. These terms may need a brief explanation.

A placebo is an inactive substance which is indistinguishable from an active substance or drug, so that any patient taking a placebo in a trial will not know whether it is the real drug or the inactive placebo. The reason for using placebos is that some people are psychologically susceptible to the suggestion that a substance, believed to be a beneficial drug, will improve their condition, and this belief may be so strong as to make them actually feel better or even produce a measurable physical improvement. It is very dangerous, therefore, to attempt to evaluate a drug by giving it on its own to patients, many of whom will desperately want to feel better, some perhaps just to please the doctor who is giving them the drug. In a placebo-controlled trial, half the subjects will be given the drug and half will be given a placebo, indistinguishable from the drug. Any observed differences in the results between the drug and placebo group must therefore be due to the drug and not to the general placebo effect.

The double-blind factor refers to a trial where neither the patients nor the researchers know (until the end of the trial) which of the subjects are taking the drug and which the placebo. This prevents researchers who may have spent months developing a drug from recording results more favourably in respect of subjects in the drug group. As explained in chapter 8, the group who receive the therapeutic agent rather than the placebo are often referred to as the *verum* group.

Some trials involve the testing of drugs on animals in laboratories. There are ethical and moral issues surrounding such testings. The author is of the opinion that in the case of garlic and ginkgo, both of which are natural products which have been used as medicines (and, in the case of garlic, as food) for thousands of years, clinical trials involving human volunteers are the most valuable method of assessing the medical benefit of the two plants for treating diseases in humans. Accordingly, none of the trials discussed below involve the use of live animals.

The trials selected are all from recent refereed journals and are believed to be reasonably sound in the methodology used. Should the reader want to refer to the original papers, full references are given at the end of the book.

After the summary of the trials there may be additional comments by this author to highlight any points of particular interest or to expand on any topic raised in the trial.

TRIALS ASSESSING THE EFFECT OF GARLIC AGAINST FACTORS PREDISPOSING DISEASES OF THE CIRCULATORY SYSTEM

Effect of dried garlic on blood coagulation, fibrinolysis, platelet aggregation and serum cholesterol levels in patients with hyperlipoproteinaemia
J. Harenberg, C. Giese and R. Zimmerman

A study carried out by the Medical Clinic of the University of Heidelberg in 1988 looked at the effect of dried garlic on the blood coagulation, fibrinolysis, platelet aggregation and serum cholesterol levels in patients with hyperlipoproteinaemia. Twenty patients were chosen with hyperlipoproteinaemia and hypercholesterolaemia, all of whom had coronary artery disease and seventeen of whom had previously experienced myocardial infarction. Doses of 600mg (3 × 200mg) of dried garlic were given each day to each patient over a period of four weeks with no other modifications to their diet.

Blood tests at the end of the trial showed the following results:

Serum cholesterol levels	7.1% average reduction
Serum fibrinogen levels	10.0% average reduction
Systolic blood pressure	8.1% average reduction
Serum platelet aggregating factor	no significant reduction

Levels of fibrinopeptide (FpB b 15–42) increased during the trial, indicating that garlic is responsible for activating plasminogen which cleaves fibrin in human blood.

Comment. *A relatively short-term trial (four weeks) showed a 7 per cent reduction in serum cholesterol and an 8 per cent reduction in blood pressure. Both of these factors would be of benefit to anyone with a disease of the circulation. A 10 per cent reduction in the serum levels of fibrinogen, a factor in blood-clotting, would be beneficial to anyone susceptible to thrombosis. Fibrinogen is a large plasma protein which is converted into fibrin, the threadlike matrix which traps blood cells in the clotting process. It would appear that the mechanism by which garlic reduces the level of fibrinogen is via the activation of plasminogen, a fibrinolytic (fibrin-splitting) enzyme which removes inappropriate clots by breaking down the fibrin which holds the clot together.*

Can garlic reduce levels of serum lipids? A controlled clinical study
K. Adesh, et al.

A controlled clinical study was carried out in 1993 at the Clinical Research Centre of the Tulane University School of Medicine in New Orleans, Louisiana, to assess the effect of garlic on serum lipids. Forty-two otherwise healthy volunteers but with high serum total cholesterol levels of 220mg/100cm^3 or above were given either a placebo or 300mg garlic powder in capsule form, three times a day. The trial was 'double-blind', so neither the volunteers nor the researchers knew who was receiving the placebo or who was receiving the garlic. The trial lasted a total of twelve weeks. The results were as follows:

Placebo	serum cholesterol before	276 mg/100cm^3
	serum cholesterol after	274 mg/100cm^3
	change (decrease)	-0.10%

	LDL-cholesterol before	191 mg/100cm^3
	LDL-cholesterol after	185 mg/100cm^3
	change (decrease)	-3.2%
Garlic	serum cholesterol before	262 mg/100cm^3
	serum cholesterol after	248 mg/100cm^3
	change (decrease)	-5.65%
	LDL-cholesterol before	188 mg/100cm^3
	LDL-cholesterol after	168 mg/100cm^3
	change (decrease)	-11.90%

No significant changes between either the placebo or garlic group were noted for blood pressure or HDL-cholesterol levels.

Comment. *The placebo group remained virtually unchanged during the study, so the reduction in the level of cholesterol in the blood of the other group could only be attributable to the regular doses of garlic. The reduction in LDL-cholesterol would appear to indicate that the garlic is inhibiting the production of LDL carriers in the liver. Both the decrease in serum cholesterol and LDL-cholesterol would be of benefit to anyone susceptible to circulatory diseases involving atheroma.*

Garlic, onions and cardiovascular risk factors. A review of the evidence from human experiments with emphasis on commercially available preparations
J. Kleijnen, P. Knipschild and G. Terriet

This paper, published in 1989, was a review of other papers published on trials of garlic (and onions) to determine their effect on serum lipids and blood-clotting factors. They criticised the methodology of many of the trials and concluded that further research was necessary to establish the true effectiveness of garlic in the treatment or prevention of cardiovascular disease. It appeared that the effectiveness of commercial preparations of garlic produced the most contradictory results and concluded: 'The results of the experiments with fresh garlic are consistent: garlic causes an increase of fibrinolytic activity, it inhibits platelet aggregation and it also lowers cholesterol levels.'

Effect of garlic on platelet aggregation in patients with increased risk of juvenile ischaemic attack
H. Kiesewetter et al.

This double-blind, placebo-controlled study, conducted in 1993 by the University of the Saarland in Germany, tested the effect of garlic on platelet aggregation in people with cerebrovascular risk factors. The verum group received 800mg of powdered garlic each day for four weeks, which led to 56.3 per cent decrease in spontaneous platelet aggregation with no significant change occurring in the placebo group. The ratio of circulating platelet aggregates also decreased by 10.3 per cent, and although levels of both these factors returned to normal four weeks after the trial, the research indicates that garlic could prove useful in preventing diseases associated with platelet aggregation.

The actions of garlic referred to above are also confirmed in the following recent research papers:

Consumption of a garlic clove a day could be beneficial in preventing thrombosis. *M. Ali and M. Thomson, 1994.*

Effect of garlic and fish-oil supplementation on serum lipid and lipoprotein concentrations in hypercholesterolaemic men. *A. J. Adler and B. J. Holub,* 1997.

Garlic powder in the treatment of moderate hyperlipidaemia: a controlled trial and meta-analysis. *H. A. Neil et al.,* 1996.

A double-blind crossover study in moderately hypercholesterolaemic men that compared the effect of aged garlic extract and placebo administration on blood lipids. *M. Steiner, A. H. Khan, D. Holbert and R. I. Lin,* 1996.

COMBINED TRIALS OF GINKGO AND GARLIC

Limitation of the deterioration of lipid parameters by a standardised garlic-ginkgo combination product. A multicenter placebo-controlled double-blind study
R. Kenzelmann and F. Kade

This is perhaps the only trial to assess the effect of garlic and ginkgo together for the treatment of hyperlipidaemia. The product used was called 'Allium plus' and the indications are that the garlic content was the main agent under investigation. The investigation was a two-month randomised placebo-controlled double-blind study over the Christmas and New Year period of 1992–3, when the lipid intake was anticipated to be high. The trial showed that the subjects who took 'Allium plus' had significantly less serum cholesterol at the end of the study than did the placebo group. Interestingly, a follow-up analysis, eight weeks after both groups had ceased to take any antihyperlipidaemic agent, showed that their serum cholesterol levels had returned to the levels existing before the trial began.

Comment. *The problem with this trial is that it does not differentiate between the effects of garlic and ginkgo on cholesterol levels. It would have been useful to have had a garlic only and a ginkgo only group so that it could have been established which agent was giving the therapeutic effect and whether there was any synergistic action when garlic and ginkgo are used together. The fact that cholesterol levels returned to normal when medication ceased shows the need for patients to maintain the dosage long term.*

TRIALS ASSESSING THE EFFECT OF GINKGO BILOBA EXTRACTS ON FACTORS PREDISPOSING CARDIOVASCULAR DISEASE

Hemorheologic effects of *Ginkgo biloba* extract EGb 761. Dose-dependent effect of EGb 761 on microcirculation and viscoelasticity of blood
P. Koltringer et al.

This 1993 German research trial looked at the effect of EGb 761 (Tebonin) on the viscosity of the blood using Doppler flowmetry to evaluate microcirculation in the skin. Forty-two patients were used in the trial, all of whom had pathological blood visco-elasticity values, and it was found that the ginkgo extract reduced the blood viscosity with its effect increasing with dosage.

Comment. *The more viscous, or 'thicker' the blood, the greater will be the resistance in the peripheral capillaries and the more pressure will be required to push the blood through the capillaries. A reduction in the viscosity of the blood could assist in the reduction of blood pressure in certain cases.*

TRIALS ASSESSING THE EFFECT OF *GINKGO BILOBA* EXTRACTS IN THE TREATMENT OF CEREBRAL INSUFFICIENCY

In the West, the most frequent medical use of *Ginkgo biloba* is in the treatment of idiopathic cerebral insufficiency in the elderly. Prescription is generally in the form of standardised extracts, especially EGb 761, marketed under trade names such as Tebonin® and Tanakan®. The use of ginkgo by orthodox practitioners is almost exclusive to continental Europe, especially Germany where over five million prescriptions are issued each year at a cost of more than 300 million DM. In the UK, the use of ginkgo by the orthodox medical profession is almost unknown. It should be of little surprise, therefore, that most of the trials of ginkgo have taken place on the continent, but the author has selected two of the few trials of ginkgo conducted in the UK which are included amongst those described below.

A double-blind placebo-based trial of *Tanakan* in the treatment of idiopathic cognitive impairment in the elderly
K. Wesnes et al.

This trial took place in the Kent area of the UK in 1987. It was designed to test the effect of a commercially prepared extract of *Ginkgo biloba* called *Tanakan* on the mental efficiency and quality of life of a selected group of 58 elderly patients suffering from a mild impairment of their mental functions. Patients suffering from clinical dementia were excluded, as were those patients suffering from a predisposing cause for their symptoms such as a metabolic or endocrine imbalance, infection, neurological disorder, etc. The subjects were randomly allocated to a placebo group or a *Tanakan* group which received 40mg of *Tanakan* taken three times each day for 12 weeks. During this period a series of clinically recognised cognitive tests were performed to assess the progress of the subjects. The tests assessed included the ability of subjects to memorise words and numbers under controlled conditions.

The results produced were too complex to be replicated here, but they were analysed using standard techniques and statistical methods. In all of the eight tests performed by the patients, there was an improvement in performance for the *Tanakan* group compared to the placebo group, especially in the latter part of the study. Both the speed and accuracy of mental processing of the *Tanakan* group improved compared with the placebo group and the *Tanakan* group also reported an increase in their degree of interest in everyday life.

The researchers concluded that *Tanakan* would be useful in the treatment of patients in the early stages of primary generative dementia.

Clinical notes. *The processes which cause damage to the brain after ischaemic attacks are not well understood, but the theory now most widely accepted is that the surge of oxygen-rich blood* *to ischaemic areas (reperfusion) causes most of the damage. This increase in brain oxygen may trigger the formation of platelet activating factor (PAF), leading to inflammation and free radical formation, along with various metabolites of arachidonic acid. Ginkgolides are recognised PAF antagonists and their presence in the brain during reperfusion may attenuate the formation of PAF, and reduce inflammation and the resulting superoxide free radicals.*

Effect of LI 1370 to help patients with cerebral insufficiency. A multi-centre, double blind study by the German Association of General Practitioners
E. Bruchert et al.

In a double-blind, placebo-controlled trial in 1991, controlled by the German Association of General Practitioners, 209 outpatients, selected for cerebral insufficiency, were given either 150mg doses of Kaveri (LI 1370), a commercial ginkgo extract, or a placebo each day for twelve weeks. Twelve symptoms relating to cerebral insufficiency were assessed and for eight of the symptoms, a significant difference was established between improvements experienced by the ginkgo and placebo group. Although patients in both groups reported feeling better for the treatment, clinical assessment showed the greatest measurable improvement had occurred in the ginkgo group.

patients reporting an improvement	ginkgo	83 per cent
patients reporting an improvement	placebo	53 per cent
clinical confirmation of improvement	ginkgo	71 per cent
clinical confirmation of improvement	placebo	32 per cent

Comment. *The marked improvement in the patients receiving ginkgo concurs with other trials. However, note should be taken of the significant improvement, both perceived and clinically measured, in the placebo group. This shows the power of the placebo effect and the necessity for placebo control. For example, if a new drug believed to be of therapeutic value but in fact inert was tested using a non-placebo trial, then a clinical improvement* *of 32 per cent could have led the researchers to believe that the drug was of significant therapeutic value. However, with a placebo control, the improvement is negated and the drug is shown to have no therapeutic value.*

The action of ginkgo extract in the treatment of cerebral insufficiency is also confirmed in the following research papers:

Ginkgo biloba for cerebral insufficiency. *J. Kleijnen and P. Knipschild*, 1992.

A double-blind, placebo-controlled study of *Ginkgo biloba* extract ('Tanakan') in elderly outpatients with mild to moderate memory impairment. *G. S. Rai, C. Shovlin and K. A. Wesnes*, 1991.

TRIALS ASSESSING THE EFFECT OF *GINKGO BILOBA* EXTRACTS IN THE TREATMENT OF DEAFNESS AND TINNITUS

Ginkgo extract EGb 761 (Tenobin)/HAES versus naftidrofuryl (Dusodril)/HAES. A randomised study of therapy of sudden deafness
F. Hoffmann, C. Beck, A. Schutz and P. Offermann

The 1994 research compared the efficacy of EGb 761 (Tebonin) with a regularly prescribed vasodilatory drug, naftidrofuryl (Dusodril) in treating idiopathic (ie. cause unknown) sudden deafness. Eighty patients were randomly selected to receive either EGb 761 or naftidrofuryl for three weeks. After allowing for cases of spontaneous remission, the EGb 761 was shown to be marginally more effective than naftidrofuryl and without any of the associated side-effects.

Comments. *The mechanisms of actions of the ginkgo extract and naftidrofuryl are somewhat similar in that they are both vasodilators, but EGb 761 also has free radical scavenging properties and is a platelet activating factor antagonist. The increased* *effectiveness of ginkgo may be due to the wider range of thera-peutic actions.*

Can vestibular compensation be enhanced by drug treatment? A review of recent evidence
P. F. Smith and C. L. Darlington

This review in 1994 analysed published reports on the efficacy of various types of drug in treating unilateral vestibular deafferentation (UVD) which causes ocular, motor and postural disorders. Recovery from this disorder is often by vestibular compensation and the authors concluded that there was good evidence that the ginkgo extract EGb 761 (together with melanotropic peptides) accelerated the recovery process.

TRIALS ASSESSING THE EFFECT OF *GINKGO BILOBA* EXTRACTS IN THE TREATMENT OF INTERMITTENT CLAUDICATION

Placebo-controlled double-blind study of the effectiveness of *Ginkgo biloba* special extract EGb 761 in trained patients with intermittent claudication
J. Blume, M. Kieser and U. Holscher

In this placebo-controlled, randomised, double-blind study, conducted in 1996, the effect of the *Ginkgo biloba* extract EGb 761 was assessed on the walking performance of patients suffering from intermittent claudication. Forty-two men, aged 47–82 years, with peripheral arterial occlusive disease of the lower extremities and intermittent claudication, were recruited to the study, none of whom could walk farther than 150 metres on a treadmill. The group was randomly divided into EGb 761 and placebo, the former being given 40mg of EGb 761 three times each day and the latter an indistinguishable placebo. The effects of the treatment were assessed after 8, 16 and 24 weeks and the researchers found that the *Ginkgo biloba* extract EGb 761 produced a statistically significant and clinically relevant improvement of the walking performance in the patients, with little evidence of side-effects. The patients receiving EGb 761 increased their pain-free walking distance by an average of 34 metres compared to an increase of 8 metres for the placebo group.

Study of the anti-ischaemic action of EGb 761 in the treatment of peripheral arterial occlusive disease by TcPO$_2$ determination
X. Mouren, P. Caillard and F. Schwartz

This randomised, placebo-controlled, double-blind research in 1994 assessed the anti-ischaemic effect of *Ginkgo biloba* extract EGb 761 by measuring the amount of oxygen in the peripheral blood circulation during exercise, using non-invasive transcutaneous oximetry. Twenty patients suffering from claudicating atherosclerotic arterial occlusive disease and aged between 44 and 73 years were given either a placebo or 320mg of EGb 761 each day for four weeks. In the EGb 761 group the areas of ischaemia decreased by 38 per cent but remained stable (+5 per cent) in the placebo group.

TRIALS ASSESSING THE EFFECT OF *GINKGO BILOBA* EXTRACTS IN THE TREATMENT OF PREMENSTRUAL PROBLEMS

Value of standardised *Ginkgo biloba* extract (EGb 761) in the management of congestive symptoms of premenstrual syndrome
A. Tamborini and R. Taurelle

In this 1993 French study, 165 women between the ages of 18 and 45, suffering from congestive premenstrual problems, were given either a placebo or the *Ginkgo biloba* extract EGb 761 from the sixteenth day of one cycle until the fifth day of the next cycle. The researchers found that the women taking the ginkgo extract showed a significant improvement in symptoms of a physical and neurophysiological nature. Congestive symptoms associated with the breasts were particularly improved.

ADDITIONAL RESEARCH RELATING TO THE ACTIONS OF GARLIC AND GINKGO AS THERAPEUTIC AGENTS

So far we have looked at those trials which have examined the effects of garlic and ginkgo on patients. The traditional actions of both of these plants have been confirmed scientifically: garlic has a beneficial effect in the treatment of cardiovascular disease and ginkgo is useful in the treatment of cerebral insufficiency. Although clinical trials are the ultimate test of a therapeutic agent's usefulness, often they do not give us much information about how the agent works. This is where laboratory experiments are useful, especially when we are looking at the actions of a particular substance at a biochemical or a cellular level.

GARLIC—RESEARCH RELATING TO ITS THERAPEUTIC ACTIONS

Garlic reduces plasma lipids by inhibiting hepatic cholesterol and triacylglycerol synthesis
Y. Y. Yeh and S. M. Yeh

This research, carried out by the Pennsylvania State University in 1994, used water and alcohol extracts of fresh garlic to determine the mechanism whereby garlic reduces serum cholesterol and serum triglycerides. They found that garlic inhibits the production of cholesterol in the liver and the triacylglycerol levels were lowered by the inhibition of fatty acid synthesis.

Effect of ajoene, the major antiplatelet compound from garlic, on platelet thrombus action
R. Apitz-Castro, J. Badimon and L. Badimon

This research, conducted at the Massachusetts General Hospital and Harvard Medical School in 1992, looked at the effect of ajoene, a metabolite secondary to the oxidation of alliin, produced when garlic is crushed. It measured the effect of ajoene on platelet deposition on isolated endothelium tissue such as that found in the lining of the arteries. Ajoene was found to significantly reduce the level of platelet aggregation and also inhibited the binding of fibrinogen, the soluble plasma protein which on conversion to fibrin is responsible for enmeshing the blood cells in clot formation.

Ajoene, the antiplatelet principle of garlic, synergistically potentiates the anti-aggregatory action of prostacyclin, forskolin, indomethacin and dypiridamole on human platelets
R. Apitz-Castro, R. Vargas and M. Jain

In normal, undamaged blood vessels the tendency for platelets to aggregate is resisted by a potent anti-aggregatory chemical called prostacyclin which is secreted by the endothelial cells that line the blood vessels. This 1996 research found that ajoene from garlic not only enhances the effectiveness of prostacyclin itself, but also works synergistically to improve the performance of the anticoagulatory drugs mentioned in the title of the paper.

Potent activation of nitric oxide synthase by garlic: a basis for its therapeutic applications
I. Das, N. S. Khan and S. R. Sooranna

This research by the Charing Cross and Westminster Medical School in London, conducted in 1995, confirmed that water and alcoholic extracts of garlic are both very potent inhibitors of platelet aggregation. Dilutions of garlic extract also promoted nitric oxide synthase activity in isolated platelets *in vitro* and in placental villous tissue. Nitric oxide is now believed to be an important anti-clotting mediator produced by healthy blood vessels.

Effects of garlic extract and of three pure components isolated from it on human platelet aggregation, arachidonate metabolism, release reaction and platelet ultrastructure
R. Apitz-Castro et al.

In this 1993 study, three pure substances were isolated from fresh garlic and tested on human platelet aggregation, arachidonate metabolism, release reaction and platelet ultrastructure. The researchers found that all of the substances inhibited platelet aggregation, but one, designated F3 and putatively identified as 1, 5-hexadienyltrisulfide, was the most potent anti-aggregant by a factor of four, and that its effect lasted for over three hours after treatment. The researchers also found that F3 inhibited the thrombin-induced release of ATP and that arachidonate metabolism was reduced.

The actions of garlic referred to above are also confirmed in the following research papers:

Evaluation of hydroxyl radical-scavenging property of garlic. *K. Prasad, V. A. Laxdal, M. Yu and B. L. Raney*, 1996.

Effects of a garlic-derived principle (ajoene) on aggregation and arachidonic acid metabolism in human blood platelets. *K. C. Srivastava and O. D. Tyagi*, 1993.

GINKGO—RESEARCH RELATING TO ITS THERAPEUTIC ACTIONS

Comparison of three PAF-acether receptor antagonist ginkgolides
R. Korth, D. Nunez, J. Bidault and J. Benveniste

This research study, at the Paris South University in France in 1988, looked at the effect of various ginkgolides on platelets and platelet aggregation. It found that of the ginkgolides tested, BN5021 was the most effective in the inhibition of platelet aggregation and also in the binding of platelet activating factor to human platelets. The researchers concluded that ginkgolides work by binding to PAF receptors on the platelets, thus blocking activation by PAF and so inhibiting platelet aggregation. In an adjunct to the research they reported that the oral administration of one of the ginkgolides, (52063) caused an inhibition to the inflammatory response in healthy volunteers induced by the subcutaneous injection of PAF.

Hydroxyl and superoxide anion radical scavenging activities of natural source antioxidants using the computerised JES-FR30 ESR spectrometer system
Y. Noda et al.

The free radical scavenging activities of various water soluble plant extracts, including *Ginkgo biloba* (in the extract form EGb 761), were examined by researchers at the University of California, Berkeley, in 1997, using electron spin resonance spectroscopy. The results showed that for the superoxide anion (O·), *Ginkgo biloba* had the greatest scavenging activity, but that green tea and pine bark extract had the greatest hydroxyl (OH) free radical scavenging ability, followed creditably close by *Ginkgo biloba*.

The neuroprotective properties of the *Ginkgo biloba* leaf: a review of the possible relationship to platelet-activating factor (PAF)
P. F. Smith, K. Maclennan and C. L. Darlington

In this review article published in 1996, the authors concluded, 'There is substantial experimental evidence to support the view that *Ginkgo biloba* extracts have neuroprotective properties under conditions such as hypoxia/ischaemia, seizure activity and peripheral nerve damage. One of the components of *Ginkgo biloba*, ginkgolide B, is a potent platelet-activating factor (PAF) antagonist. Although the terpene fraction of *Ginkgo biloba*, which contains the ginkgolides, may contribute to the neuroprotective properties of the *Ginkgo biloba* leaf, it is also likely that the flavonoid fraction, containing free radical scavengers, is important in this respect.'

The Chemistry of Cholesterol

In this book we have looked at cholesterol in general terms, what it does and how you can reduce your levels of cholesterol by dietary changes. Here we examine cholesterol in more detail, look at its functions and chemistry and explain the mechanism whereby it contributes to the formation of atheromatous plaques in the arteries.

Cholesterol is a lipid found abundantly in all the *cell membranes* of all the cells of all animals. It is important for stabilising the cell membrane, and without its presence the membrane would not perform its function of regulating the movement of substances in and out of the cell. The percentage of cholesterol in the various membranes varies but is typically around 20 per cent of the total lipid mass.

Cholesterol is also an important precursor (building block) for steroid hormones such as *androgens, oestrogens, progestogens, mineralocorticoids* and *glucocorticoids*. These hormones have important functions in the body, including the regulation of blood pressure, electrolyte balance, stress reaction, blood sugar metabolism, reproductive cycles and the maintenance of secondary sexual characteristics. Figure 11 shows the similarity between the cholesterol molecule and that of *oestradiol*, the principal ovarian oestrogen.

Cholesterol is also a precursor of *vitamin D* which is essential for the absorption of calcium and proper bone formation. Although vitamin D is usually obtained from dietary sources, it can also be synthesised in the body when skin is exposed to ultra violet radiation from the sun. In this case *7-dehydrocholesterol* is transformed into *previtamin D* and then into *vitamin D_3*.

Figure 11   Similarities in structure between cholesterol and oestradiol (oestrogen)

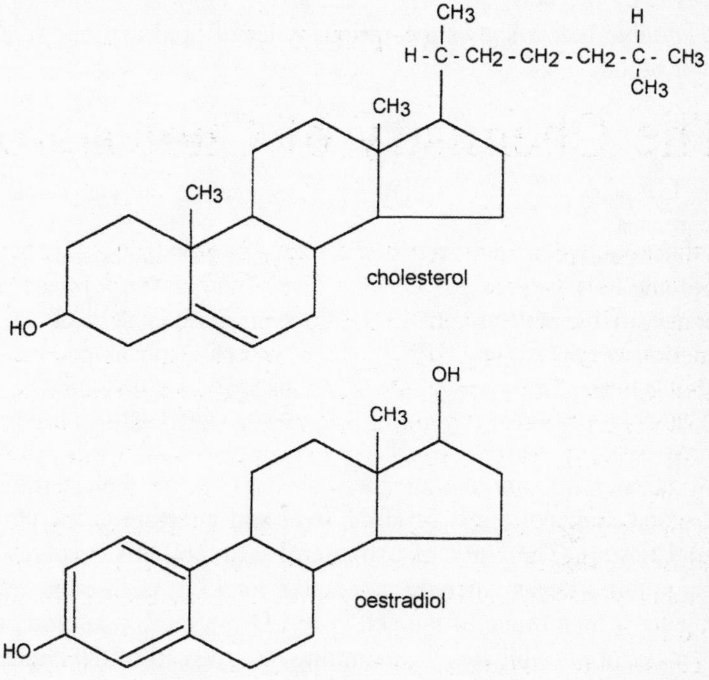

cholesterol

oestradiol

As with all lipids, cholesterol is highly hydrophobic (it is repelled by water) and does not mix readily with water. A special, and rather complex mechanism is therefore needed for the transport of cholesterol in the watery medium of the blood. This is done by various special carrier structures, called *chylomicrons* and *lipoproteins*, made up, as the name of the latter suggests, of lipids and proteins. These minute globular structures have a surface structure which makes then soluble in blood, the cholesterol being kept separate from the blood within the core of the carrier. The nomenclature of many of the carriers relates to their ratio of protein to lipid. Thus, very low density lipoproteins (VLDLs) have very little protein (and more lipid which is lighter) whilst high density lipoproteins (HDLs) contain a large amount of protein and a correspondingly smaller proportion of lipid. Some of these carriers carry lipids of dietary origin and others carry those lipids synthesised by the body.

The table below shows the various types of lipid carriers found in the blood.

Name	abbreviation	lipid carried
Very low density lipoproteins	VLDL	synthesised triacylglycerols
Intermediate density lipoproteins	IDL	synthesised cholesterol
Low density lipoproteins	LDL	synthesised cholesterol
High density lipoproteins	HDL	synthesised cholesterol
Chylomicrons	-	dietary triacylglycerols
Chylomicron remnants	-	dietary cholesterol

Low density lipoproteins are the main carriers of cholesterol in the blood, transporting it from the liver and intestine to the peripheral tissues. The entry of cholesterol into the cells involves a recognition process whereby a receptor for LDL is inserted into the plasma membrane of the cell. The LDL in the blood binds to this receptor and initiates the engulfing into the cell of the cholesterol within the LDL shell. This engulfing process is called *endocytosis*. Tissues needing to increase their uptake of cholesterol synthesise new receptor sites which bind to more LDL.

The normal concentration of cholesterol in the blood is around 300mg per 1000ml, and if there is insufficient supply of cholesterol in the diet then up to 800mg each day can be synthesised in the liver and intestines. The synthesis of cholesterol is regulated by the supply of dietary cholesterol suppressing the enzyme *3 hydroxy, 3 methylglutaryl CoA reductase* which catalyses the formation of *mevalonate*, a stage in the biosynthesis of cholesterol. It can be seen that the reduction of plasma cholesterol levels by dietary control is not straightforward, because as less is consumed in the diet, so the production of endogenous cholesterol in the liver is increased to compensate.

High density lipoproteins are responsible for scavenging the tissue cells for excess cholesterol released from damaged cells and from the debris of old cells undergoing the normal processes of replacement. One of the proteins on the surface of HDL is a co-factor for the plasma enzyme *lecithin cholesterol acetyl transferase* (LCAT), which esterifies cholesterol, thus making it even more hydrophobic and inducing its transfer to the core of the HDL, so removing cholesterol from the plasma.

Excess cholesterol arriving at the liver is secreted in the bile, either as bile salts or as cholesterol. The bile leaves the liver via the bile duct, empties into the duodenum and is eventually excreted. It should be noted that the cholesterol in the bile salts plays an important part in the emulsification of dietary fat in the processes of digestion.

It has been unequivocally shown that high plasma cholesterol levels predispose individuals to atherosclerosis and its associated diseases. For those without specific metabolic malfunctions of the cholesterol regulatory system, dietary control should be sufficient to maintain appropriate levels of cholesterol. Eating habits, involving an excess consumption of foods rich in cholesterol and triacylglycerols, overload the internal regulatory system, tissue cell cholesterol receptors are suppressed and regulation then depends on receptor independent mechanisms which are less well understood. Some of the excess cholesterol is accumulated in scavenging macrophages which may result in lipid deposition in arterial walls. It has been estimated that up to 50 per cent of the population of Britain may be clinically defined as having *hyperlipoproteinaemia*, primarily due to an injudicious diet. A small proportion of those mentioned above may have metabolic disorders involving receptor or enzyme deficiency, which may not respond solely to a change in diet.

The plasma levels of cholesterol predisposing an individual to circulatory disease need to be considered in terms of the HDL: total plasma cholesterol ratio. The main factor which increases HDL levels appears to be exercise, whilst smoking depresses them. Unsaturated fats appear to stimulate the elimination of cholesterol and bile salts by the liver, and both oats and psyllium husks prevent the absorption of cholesterol from the gut. There is also evidence of oestrogen conferring some protection against heart disease: HDL levels are lower in pre-menopausal women, whereas after the menopause the incidence of circulatory disorders in women is similar to that of men.

Herbs Ancient and Modern

Ever since *Homo sapiens* evolved, plants have formed a large component of human diet. As people tried eating different plants they would have learnt which tasted good, which helped them to recover from various illnesses, and which few would poison them.

Thus every human culture, at every stage in its history, used some form of herbal medicine. Remains of medicinal plants have been found in ancient burial mounds, and some of the world's earliest books, from China and Egypt, include information on the use of plant medicines.

The great civilisations of early China would have been familiar with the ginkgo tree. Their written accounts of the use of herbal medicines date back more than 4,000 years. The practice of medicine developed quite differently in China from that of the West, in that the theories developed by scholars were not put into practice by them: the actual work of treating disease was considered too lowly, and was more the work of an artisan than an intellectual. The Chinese world view was reflected in the medical systems they devised, and although these have gone through great changes over the centuries, herbal medicine still has an accepted place in China, alongside modern drug therapy and, of course, acupuncture.

In other less developed parts of the world medical knowledge was often passed on from generation to generation, in families who had special status as healers or wise men and women. This pattern is still found among tribal peoples who have had limited contact with the outside world. Although most people in the tribe would know something of healing plants, the 'specialists' were called in to treat any serious health problems.

As civilisation developed in the West, the Greeks became the pioneers in medicine as they were in so many other arts and sciences. Later, during the Roman Empire, herbal medicine flourished. United under the rule of the Empire, doctors and healers from places as far apart as Britain, North Africa and the Near East came into contact for the first time. Medical practice took great strides forward, and new books were written that remained standard texts for hundreds of years. Following the decline of the Empire, the Christian monks of Europe and the scholars of the Islamic world maintained the skills, but still looked back to the Greeks and Romans as the source of medical authority.

After the voyages of discovery in the fifteenth and sixteenth centuries, to both the New World and the East, a wealth of new plants was introduced into Europe. There was always hope that these would provide cures for the devastating epidemic diseases of the time (garlic was one of those favoured as a prevention against the plague) and many wealthy families' fortunes were based on the importation of costly exotic herbs and spices. The discoveries also stimulated a new, forward-looking spirit of investigation into the natural world, which dared to challenge the authority of the ancient academic texts.

With the rise of science in Europe, new chemical remedies, prescribed by university-trained doctors, became far more popular with the wealthy than the 'old-fashioned' herbs. The price they paid often turned out to be greater than the money involved, for many of the chemicals, such as arsenic and antimony, were highly toxic. Herbal medicine became associated with those who could only afford the services of the local wise woman whose medicines grew freely in the woods and meadows. In spite of its known efficacy, in Tudor times garlic was despised as a remedy of the 'vulgar poor', limiting the value that doctors ascribed to it. Many innocent country people were vilified or persecuted for helping others by practising mainly harmless skills taught to them by family or friends.

Over the last hundred years herbal medicine has undergone great changes in its popularity and acceptability, with both doctors and the general public. At the start of the twentieth century there were still many diseases for which no type of medicine had a successful treatment. Epidemics killed thousands of people and were aggravated by conditions of poverty and poor sanitation. Herbal medicines often had as good a rate of success with these diseases as the orthodox approach.

Despite the efforts of some dedicated supporters of herbal medicine in the nineteenth century, who had mostly tried to combine the natural with the scientific approach in their studies and practice, the profile of herbal medicine declined, reaching an all-time low in the United Kingdom during the 1940s. Herbal practitioners were effectively outlawed, and continued their work under the threat of legal prosecution. With scientific developments in analytical and manufacturing techniques, the pharmaceuticals industry flourished. The treatment of infections was revolutionised by the discovery of antibiotics (penicillin itself is derived from a natural fungus— mainly *Penicillium chrysogenum*) and in the 1960s the new classes of tranquilliser drugs related to diazepam seemed at first to solve the problems of thousands of patients. Steroid drugs appeared to cure conditions like asthma and eczema almost like magic. In comparison, herbal medicines were seen as old-fashioned: garlic was consigned to the pages of the history books. The belief of herbalists in the use of the whole plant, rather than just isolated 'active constituents', met with little sympathy from orthodox doctors who saw plants only as a crude source of medicines. Plants had to be 'purified' to make medicines, such as quinine, used in the treatment of malaria, which was extracted from the South American cinchona tree. The National Health Service meant that a doctor's services were available to all, so that knowledge about self-treatment with plants which had previously been in common use was neglected. By the 1960s only a few dedicated herbalists were left, and they had to mount a tireless campaign to regain the legal right to practise (granted in the 1968 Medicines Act).

But the climate of opinion started to change as the public became increasingly disillusioned with orthodox medicines. 'Wonder' drugs were found to have side-effects: antibiotics risk the development of resistant 'superbugs'; the overuse of tranquillisers leads to dependency and long-term side-effects, and prolonged steroid use can bring problems like weight-gain and osteoporosis. Industrial processes were found to cause pollution, high-tech living produced unexpected stresses, and people wanted to feel more in harmony with the natural world. More people, including myself, were becoming interested in learning the skills of the herbal practitioners, and the number of qualified herbalists began to increase.

Scientists are now becoming more open-minded about what herbs have to offer: a new appreciation that the 'single active constituent' approach might be inappropriate for investigating herbal medicines is developing. At present the growth of research is enormous, confirming the benefits of many of the traditional remedies and revealing many new properties and uses. Current work is scientifically 'respectable', being carried out according to conventional scientific method. The results are undoubtedly valid, and are being accepted by orthodox scientists and doctors in a way that would have been undreamt of twenty years ago.

After two hundred years of being derided, herbal remedies are coming into their own as a safe and effective treatment. Garlic and ginkgo, both with a medicinal pedigree extending back thousands of years, are now of confirmed value in their potential for contributing to human health.

Contact Addresses

The main professional bodies of herbal practitioners are:

United Kingdom
The National Institute of Medical Herbalists
56 Longbrook Street, Exeter, Devon EX4 6AH.
Tel. 01392 426022

Register of Chinese Herbal Medicine
4 Glenleigh Terrace, Maidstone Road, Nettlestead,
Maidstone, Kent NE18 5EP

United States of America
The School of Phytotherapy
10401 Montgomery Parkway NE, Albuquerque,
New Mexico 87111.
Tel. (505) 275 0620.

Ginkgo and garlic supplies are available by mail order from:

The Herbal Apothecary
103 High Street, Syston, Leicester LE7 8GQ.
Tel. 0116 260690

References

1 Adesh, K. *et al.* Can garlic reduce levels of serum lipids? A controlled clinical study, *American Journal of Medicine*, 1993, 94: 632–635.

2 Ali, M. Mechanism by which garlic (*Allium sativum*) inhibits cyclo-oxygenase activity. Effect of raw versus boiled garlic extract on the synthesis of prostanoids, *Prostaglandins, Leukotrienes and Essential Fatty Acids*, 1995, 53(6): 397–400.

3 Ali, M. and Thomson, M. Consumption of a garlic clove a day could be beneficial in preventing thrombosis, *Prostaglandins, Leukotrienes and Essential Fatty Acids*, 1994, 53: 211–212.

4 Adler, A. J. and Holub, B. J. Effect of garlic and fish-oil supplementation on serum lipid and lipoprotein concentrations in hypercholesterolemic men, *American Journal of Clinical Nutrition*, 1997, 65(2): 445–50.

5 Apitz-Castro, R. *et al.* Effects of garlic extract and of three pure components isolated from it on human platelet aggregation, arachidonate metabolism, release reaction and platelet ultrastructure, *Thrombosis Research*, 1983, 32: 155–169.

6 Apitz-Castro, R., Vargas, R. and Jain, M. Ajoene, the antiplatelet principle of garlic, synergistically potentiates the anti-aggregatory action of prostacyclin, forskolin, indomethacin and dypiridamole on human platelets, *Thrombosis Research*, 1986, 42: 303–311.

7 Apitz-Castro, R., Badimon, J. and Badimon, L. Effect of ajoene, the major antiplatelet compound from garlic, on platelet thrombus action, *Thrombosis Research*, 1992, 68: 145–155.

8 Auer, W., Eiber, A. and Hertkorn, E. Hypertension and hyperlipidaemia: garlic helps in mild cases, *British Journal of Clinical Practice*, 1990, 44 (Suppl. 69), 3–6.

9 Blume, J., Kieser, M. and Holscher, U. Placebo-controlled double-blind study of the effectiveness of *Ginkgo biloba* special extract EGb 761 in trained patients with intermittent claudication, *Vasa*, 1996, 25(3): 265–74.
Original title: Placebokontrollierte doppelblindstudie zur wirksamkeit von *Ginkgo-biloba*-spezialextrakt EGb 761 bei austrainierten ratienten mit claudicatio intermittens.

REFERENCES

10   Bruchert, E., Heinrich, S. and Ruf-Kohler, P. Effectiveness of LI 1370 for older patients with cerebral insufficiency. Multicentre double blind study by the Society of German General Practitioners, *Münchener Medizinische Wochenschrift*, 1991, 133 (Suppl. 1), S9–S14.
Original title: Wirksamkeit von LI 1370 bei alteren patienten mit hirnleistungsschwache. Multizentrische doppelblindstudie des fach-verbandes Deutscher Allgemeinarzte.

11   Chaw, S. M., Zharkikh, A., Sung, H. M., Lau, T. C. and Li, W. H. Molecular phylogeny of extant gymnosperms and seed plant evolution: analysis of nuclear 18S rRNA sequences, *Molecular Biology and Evolution*, 1997, 14(1): 56–68.

12   Chung, K. F. *et al.* Effect of a ginkgolide mixture (BN 52063) in antagonising skin and platelet responses to platelet activating factor in man, *Lancet*, 1987, i: 248–251.

13   Das, I., Khan, N. S. and Sooranna, S. R. Potent activation of nitric oxide synthase by garlic: a basis for its therapeutic applications, *Current Medical Research and Opinion*, 1995, 13(5): 257–63.

14   Harenberg, J., Giese, C. and Zimmerman, R. Effect of dried garlic on blood coagulation, fibrinolysis, platelet aggregation and serum cholesterol levels in patients with hyperlipoproteinemia, *Atherosclerosis*, 1988, 74: 247–249.

15   Hofferberg, B. The efficacy of EGb 761 in patients with senile dementia of the Alzheimer type, a double-blind, placebo-controlled study on different levels of investigation, *Human Psychopharmacology*, 1994, 9: 215–222.

16   Hoffmann, F., Beck, C., Schutz, A. and Offermann, P. Ginkgo extract EGb 761 (Tebonin)/HAES versus naftidrofuryl (Dusodril)/HAES. A randomised study of therapy of sudden deafness, *Laryngo-Rhino-Otologie*, 1994, 73(3): 149–52.
Original title: Ginkgoextrakt EGb 761 (Tebonin)/HAES versus Naftidrofuryl (Dusodril)/HAES. Eine randomisierte Studie zur Horsturz-therapie.

17   Holgers, K. M., Axelsson, A. and Pringle, I. *Ginkgo biloba* extract for the treatment of tinnitus, *Audiology*, 1994, 33(2): 85–92.

18   Holme, G. and Morley, J. (eds.). *PAF in Asthma*, Academic Press.

19   Ide, N., Nelson, A. B. and Lau, B. H. Aged garlic extract and its constituents inhibit Cu (2+)-induced oxidative modification of low density lipoprotein, *Planta Medica*, 1997, 63(3): 263–4.

20   Kenzelmann, R. and Kade, F. Limitation of the deterioration of lipid parameters by a standardised garlic-ginkgo combination product. A multicenter placebo-controlled double-blind study, *Arzneimittel-Forschung*, 1993, 43(9): 978–81.

21 Kiesewetter, H. *et al.* Effect of garlic on platelet aggregation in patients with increased risk of juvenile ischaemic attack, *European Journal of Clinical Pharmacology*, 1993, 45(4): 333–6.

22 Kleijnen, J. and Knipschild, P. *Ginkgo biloba* for cerebral insufficiency, *British Journal of Clinical Pharmacology*, 1992, 34: 352–358.

23 Kleijnen, J., Knipschild, P. and Terriet, G. Garlic, onions and cardiovascular risk factors. A review of the evidence from human experiments with emphasis on commercially available preparations, *British Journal of Clinical Pharmacology*, 1989, 28: 535–544.

24 Koltringer, P., Langsteger, W., Klima, G., Reisecker, F. and Eber, O. Hemorheologic effects of *Ginkgo biloba* extract EGb 761. Dose-dependent effect of EGb 761 on microcirculation and viscoelasticity of blood, *Fortschritte der Medizin*, 1993, 111(10): 170–72.
Original title: Hemorheologische Effekte des *Ginkgo-biloba*-Extrakts EGb 761. Dosisabhangige Wirkung von EGb 761 auf Mikrozirkulation und Viskoelastizitat des Blutes.

25 Korth, R., Nunez, D., Bidault, J. and Benveniste, J. Comparison of three paf-acether receptor antagonist ginkgolides, *European Journal of Pharmacology*, 1988, 152: 101–110.

26 Kramsch, D. M. Atherosclerosis progression/regression lipoprotein and vessel wall determinants, *Atherosclerosis*, 1995, 118 (suppl.), S29–S36.

27 Kurosawa, M., Yamashita, T. and Kurimoto, F. Increased levels of blood platelet-activating factor in bronchial asthmatic patients with active symptoms, *Allergy*, 1994, 49(1): 60–3.

28 Mouren, X., Caillard, P. and Schwartz, F. Study of the anti-ischemic action of EGb 761 in the treatment of peripheral arterial occlusive disease by TcPO$_2$ determination, *Angiology*, 1994, 45(6): 413–17.

29 Naganawa, R. *et al.* Inhibition of microbial growth by ajoene, a sulfur-containing compound derived from garlic, *Applied and Environmental Microbiology*, 1996, 62(11): 4238–42.

30 Navab, M. *et al.* Pathogenesis of atherosclerosis [Review], *American Journal of Cardiology*, 1995, 76(9): 18C–23C.

31 Neil, H. A. *et al.* Garlic powder in the treatment of moderate hyperlipidaemia: a controlled trial and meta-analysis, *Journal of the Royal College of Physicians of London*, 1996, 30(4): 329–34.

32 Noda, Y. *et al.* Hydroxyl and superoxide anion radical scavenging activities of natural source antioxidants using the computerised JES-FR30 ESR spectrometer system, *Biochemistry and Molecular Biology International*, 1997, 42(1): 35–44.

33 Orekhov, A. N., Tertov, W., Sobenin, I. A. and Pivovarova, E. M.

Direct anti-atherosclerosis-related effects of garlic, *Annals of Medicine*, 1995, 27(1): 63–5.

34 Page, C. P. *The Platelet in Health and Disease*. Blackwell Scientific Publications.

35 Prasad, K., Laxdal, V. A., Yu, M. and Raney, B. L. Evaluation of hydroxyl radical-scavenging property of garlic, *Molecular and Cellular Biochemistry*, 1996, 154(1): 55–63.

36 Rai, G. S., Shovlin, C. and Wesnes, K. A. A double-blind, placebo-controlled study of *Ginkgo biloba* extract ('Tanakan') in elderly outpatients with mild to moderate memory impairment, *Current Medical Research and Opinion*, 1991, 12: 350–54.

37 Silagy, C. A. and Neil, H. A. A meta-analysis of the effect of garlic on blood pressure, *Journal of Hypertension*, 1994, 12(4): 463–68.

38 Simons, L. A. *et al*. On the effect of garlic on plasma lipids and lipoproteins in mild hypercholesterolaemia, *Atherosclerosis*, 1995, 113(2): 219–25.

39 Smith, P. F. and Darlington, C. L. Can vestibular compensation be enhanced by drug treatment? A review of recent evidence, *Journal of Vestibular Research*, 1994, 4(3): 169–79.

40 Smith, P. F., Maclennan, K. and Darlington, C. L. The neuroprotective properties of the *Ginkgo biloba* leaf: a review of the possible relationship to platelet-activating factor (PAF), *Journal of Ethnopharmacology*, 1996, 50: 131–39.

41 Srivastava, K. C. and Tyagi, O. D. Effects of a garlic-derived principle (ajoene) on aggregation and arachidonic acid metabolism in human blood platelets, *Prostaglandins, Leukotrienes and Essential Fatty Acids*, 1993, 49(2): 587–95.

42 Steinberg, D. A critical look at the evidence for the oxidation of LDL in atherogenesis, *Atherosclerosis*, 1997, 131: Suppl. S5–S7.

43 Steiner, M., Khan, A. H., Holbert, D. and Lin, R. I. A double-blind crossover study in moderately hypercholesterolemic men that compared the effect of aged garlic extract and placebo administration on blood lipids, *American Journal of Clinical Nutrition*, 1996, 64(6): 866–70.

44 Steinke, B., Muller, B. and Wagner, H. Biological standardisation of ginkgo extracts, *Planta Medica*, 1993, 59(2): 155–60.

45 Tamborini, A. and Taurelle, R. Value of standardised *Ginkgo biloba* extract (EGb 761) in the management of congestive symptoms of premenstrual syndrome, *Revue Française de Gynecologie et d'Obstetrique*, 1993, 88(7–9); 447–57.
Original title: Interet de l'extrait standardise de *Ginkgo biloba* (EGb

761) dans la prise en charge des symptomes congestifs du syndrome premenstruel.

46 Tsukioka, K., Matsuzaki, M., Nakamata, M. and Kayahara, H. Increased plasma levels of platelet-activating factor (PAF) and low serum PAF acetylhydrolase (PAFAH) activity in adult patients with bronchial asthma, *Japanese Journal of Allergology*, 1993, 42(2): 167–71.

47 Warringa, R. A. *et al.* Upregulation of formyl-peptide and inter-leukin-8-induced eosinophil chemotaxis in patients with allergic asthma, *Journal of Allergy and Clinical Immunology*, 1993, 91(6): 1198–205.

48 Wesnes, K. *et al.* A double-blind placebo-based trial of *Tanakan* in the treatment of idiopathic cognitive impairment in the elderly, *Human Psychopharmacology*, 1987, 2: 159–69.

49 Yeh, Y. Y. and Yeh, S. M. Garlic reduces plasma lipids by inhibiting hepatic cholesterol and triacylglycerol synthesis, *Lipids*, 1994, 29(3): 189–93.